CLINICAL PRACTICE FOR SPEECH–LANGUAGE PATHOLOGISTS IN THE SCHOOLS

CLINICAL PRACTICE FOR SPEECH-LANGUAGE PATHOLOGISTS IN THE SCHOOLS

By

LORRAINE M. MONNIN, Ph.D.

Professor, Speech Pathology
California State University, Los Angeles
Los Angeles, California

and

KATHLEEN MURPHY PETERS, M.A.

Assistant Professor, Speech Pathology
California State University, Los Angeles
Los Angeles, California

With a Foreword by

Robert L. Douglass, Ph.D.

With a Contribution by

Dorothy McJenkin, M.A.

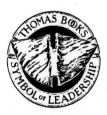

CHARLES C THOMAS • PUBLISHER
Springfield • Illinois • U.S.A.

Published and Distributed Throughout the World by
CHARLES C THOMAS • PUBLISHER
2600 South First Street
Springfield, Illinois, 62717, U.S.A.

©*1981, by* CHARLES C THOMAS • PUBLISHER
ISBN 0-398-04543-7
Library of Congress Catalog Card Number: 81-5817

*With THOMAS BOOKS careful attention is given to all details of
manufacturing and design. It is the Publisher's desire to present books
that are satisfactory as to their physical qualities and artistic possibilities
and appropriate for their particular use. THOMAS BOOKS will be
true to those laws of quality that assure a good name and good will.*

Library of Congress Cataloging in Publication Data

Monnin, Lorraine M.
   Clinical practice for speech-language pathologists in the schools.

   Bibliography: p.
   Includes index.
   1. Speech therapy for children—Study and teaching. 2. Communicative disorders in children—Study and teaching. 3. Speech therapy
for children—Study and teaching—Supervision. I. Peters, Kathleen
Murphy. II. McJenkin, Dorothy. III. Title. [DNLM: 1. Language
therapy—Education. 2. Speech pathology—Education. WV 18 M749c]
RJ496.S7M64   618.92′855′0071173   81-5817
ISBN O-398-04543-7   AACR2

Printed in the United States of America
SC-RX-1

FOREWORD

pro-fes-sion-al (adj.) One who has an assured competence in a particular field of study.

S peech-language pathology is a relatively new professional field.
It focuses on the various kinds of communication disorders that
have plagued human beings ever since human communication
began. A profession consists of an accumulated body of knowledge
and of trained and skilled persons who use that knowledge to
identify and resolve problems. For example, there are many reasons,
some obvious and some obscure, why a small child may have
problems in talking and using language. To help a child discover
the power and pleasure of communicating with others is a rich
reward for the years that a professional must devote to education
and preparation.

The training of professionals includes formal education in an
academic environment and, in a more personal way, it provides a
variety of supervised clinical experiences, which shapes a student's way of thinking about helping people. Among other things,
learning to do therapy means acquiring insight into the complex
processes involved in solving human problems. There is an orderly
approach to problem solving, beginning first with the ability to
recognize and define what the problem is, or more precisely, what
a child's individual, unique problem is. Such knowledge is not
derived solely from texts or lectures. In acquiring competence,
professionals learn to make their own observations, formulate
their own hypotheses, carry out and assess their own regimens of
therapy. The transformation of a student into a therapist occurs
during the course of deep personal involvement with human
beings struggling to communicate. It is a process of individual
exploration and discovery. Clinical training is the catalyst that
combines textbook knowledge with personal experience to produce the competent professional.

Most of the communicatively handicapped children in the United
States receive therapy within the public schools. The public school

environment poses special challenges to the professional. To function effectively, it is necessary to be knowledgeable about many things—the setting, the day-by-day operations, the roles and responsibilities of various school personnel, the sources of assistance, and the nature of the problem. The massive number of children, the hectic schedule, the uncertainties of time and space, the overwhelming paperwork, the pressures of deadlines, stand in sharp contrast to the tranquil atmosphere of the college on-campus clinic. For the student-in-training, first exposure to the public school environment can be confusing and bewildering.

It is the thesis of this text that a meaningful student teaching experience in the public schools should be carefully planned with consideration given to the roles of the student, the master clinician, and the university supervisor. The authors have experienced the public school as speech pathology students-in-training, as master clinicians, and as university supervisors. They have endeavored to map the territory, to describe the procedures for establishing clear understanding of responsibilities, and to identify the possible problems. Care and foresight in planning and clearly defined expectations should allow the student in this phase of training to receive maximum benefit from this demanding but rewarding experience.

ROBERT L. DOUGLASS

PREFACE

The public school environment poses special challenges to speech-language pathologists. For many years the public schools have been a primary employment site for students emerging from speech-language pathology training programs. Articles and books have been written on clinical supervision, and publications are available that discuss methods for implementing speech-language-hearing programs in the schools. However, there is no other book written for clinical practice in the schools that details the involvement of each member of the TRIAD.

The intent of this book is to present comprehensive information, which defines the roles and responsibilities of students, master clinicians, and university faculty involved in the training phase of speech-language pathologists for educational settings. Included is practical information on procedures relevant to training and supervising students in the schools. Guidelines and implementation procedures that give TRIAD participants a sense of direction in fulfilling requirements of the school assignment are discussed. Although the focus is the school setting, much of the information is applicable to other environments where students may be assigned for practicum experiences.

This book, like the TRIAD itself, is divided into three distinct parts: the student, the practicing speech-language pathologist, and the university faculty. To maximize the effectiveness of the TRIAD, each member has a specific role to fulfill in implementing the school practicum. By bringing this body of information together in one book, each member of the TRIAD knows his or her role and responsibilities as well as the role and responsibilities of each of the other members. This synthesizing of information makes it possible for all participants to have a broader view of the practicum experience and places each role in perspective relative to the total school experience.

Many people have generously contributed to the preparation of this book. We are grateful to the hundreds of practicing speech-language pathologists in the schools, with whom we have worked over the years, who have been so generous in making suggestions and sharing information, and to our students, on whom we field tested sections of this book.

We are particularly grateful to our families who were so patient and gave us continuous encouragement and support in this endeavor. We want to express appreciation to our colleague and friend, Patricia Klein, who so willingly shared ideas with us. We are indebted to the many speech-language pathologists who have contributed to the preparation of the manuscript. We wish to thank Jean Anderson, Katharine Butler, Sharon Iverson, James Luter, Susan Orth, Bonita Santos, Glenn Smith, Judy Snider, and Barbara Spear for their assistance.

CONTENTS

CLINICAL PRACTICE FOR

SPEECH–LANGUAGE

PATHOLOGISTS IN THE SCHOOLS

Chapter 1

THE TRIAD

A communication handicap can seriously affect a child's performance in the school environment. His performance may be below expectation, his interpersonal relationships with peers and teachers may be adversely affected, and he may be unable to develop his full potential for functioning within the academic environment. Clinical speech and language services may furnish him with skills to develop his educational capabilities. Many of these children are in regular classrooms, and a speech and language disorder is their only need for remedial services, while others are in special education classes for the educationally handicapped, learning disabled, deaf, and so forth. Speech and language remedial programs vary from state to state, but the purpose of all such programs is to help children develop their academic and social potential. In the past many children with communication handicaps have languished in classes for the mentally retarded, have dropped out of school, or have found limited opportunities for economic independence.

Since the early 1900s there has been a growing awareness of the need to serve handicapped children. In 1912, the first public school remedial speech program was begun in Detroit at the urging of concerned parents who recognized that handicapping communication disorders were impeding their children's academic progress. In the last few years there has been unprecedented activity in all areas of special education. During this time, state governments have legislated and supported special education programs in the schools. In 1977, the federal government adopted the Education for All Handicapped Children Act (PL 94-142), which mandates that all handicapped minors from ages three through twenty-one must be served through public school programs, thus assuring all children an opportunity to function in their environment.

O'Toole and Zaslow have stated, "There is no right way to

3

establish a clinical speech and hearing program in the schools. It must be tailored to the policies of the local school system, the needs of the community, and the capabilities of the staff" (1969, p. 500). Perhaps this statement best expresses the uniqueness of a school setting. The school, like a conglomerate corporation, is a sum of all its parts: state mandates, local needs, district philosophies, and personnel training. Yet, within this seeming array of diversification, school settings share a common component; the emphasis is on learning. This, then, is the setting for clinical practicum in the schools. In no way can one model be given to describe what a student assignment in the schools will encompass; however, it is the unifying component of learning that makes it possible to establish some common guidelines.

The training of a speech-language pathologist requires a solid academic background combined with comprehensive practicum experiences in various settings. An additional requirement for working in the schools is practicum experience in that environment. The on-site school experience consists of two basic components: observation of clinical practicum and student teaching.

When a college/university approves a major in speech-language pathology, it is the responsibility of the training institution to support all aspects of the program for which it has given approval. This includes support of the total curriculum and provision for faculty positions to implement the curriculum. Course work and on-campus clinical experiences are the foundation for the school assignment. A prerequisite for an effective program is that members of the speech-language pathology faculty must believe in the importance of the public school experience. They must be actively involved in the design and implementation of such a program.

In order to prepare students adequately for the school assignment, faculty need to be aware of current trends in general education as well as special education. Such knowledge of current trends in public education will allow continuous development of programs in keeping with changes in the field.

Appropriate advisement is an essential component of the program. It is necessary for students to be aware of the prerequisites and the requirements of the school assignment. The responsibilities must be so defined that students may make necessary plans. Conferring with students in advance of assignments allows for supplementary experiences that may contribute to a successful school experience.

When accepting a student, the school speech-language pathologist is making a dual commitment: (1) assuming a professional responsibility to the field and (2) defining the role of the speech-language pathologist in the school setting. Selection of speech-language pathologists should be made from those who express an interest in working with students-in-training. A student-in-training is added responsibility to the already full schedule of the speech-language pathologist, yet the satisfaction of sharing clinical skills is rewarding. Participation with training institutions can be continuing education for the on-site speech-language pathologist. Introducing students-in-training to the practicum of working in public education is a way for speech-language pathologists to reassess their own clinical techniques. They will be asked for explanations for case selection, diagnostic procedures, case history information, and so forth. They must have ready answers for the students, as well as plausible explanations for themselves.

For the students, observations provide an introduction to the school environment, and student teaching enables them to take their acquired skills into an actual work environment. It is in school settings that clinical skills are developed and broadened. Students have an opportunity to be in contact with many pupils who may be observed and assessed in an atmosphere other than a clinical setting. In no other setting is a speech-language pathologist, between 9:00 AM and 2:30 PM (forty-five minutes for lunch), expected to screen 100 first and second graders, identify those who need additional testing, select those who need remedial speech and language services, write Individualized Education Programs, work with pupils on a regular basis, and then conduct an in-service meeting from 3:00 to 5:00 PM.

Student Teaching Triad

The student teaching experience is made up of three essential components: the university supervisor, master clinician,[1] and

---

[1]At the Conference on Standards for Supervised Experience for Speech and Hearing Specialists in Public Schools (1969), the term master clinician was selected to designate the role of a speech pathologist who was assigned a student clinician.

student clinician. Each part of this TRIAD is both *intra*dependent of the other units and *inter*dependent with the other units. As in the case of a successful baseball team, each member is developing his own skills in relationship to a specific position on the team, *intra*dependency, but in order to have a winning game, each member of the team must work with the other members in a cooperative manner, *inter*dependency.

In student teaching, each of the members is *intra*dependent— each has an assignment to fulfill, each must develop individual skills, and each must demonstrate growth. The members are *inter*dependent because they recognize that alone they do not have the full concept of what is needed for successful completion of the assignment. They draw on the skills and background of the other members, and they share a common goal, which can be achieved best by working together cooperatively. A sense of well-being and self-confidence enables the members to contribute more fully to the total experience. In order to achieve the goal of developing skilled clinicians, each unit of the student teaching TRIAD must operate effectively.

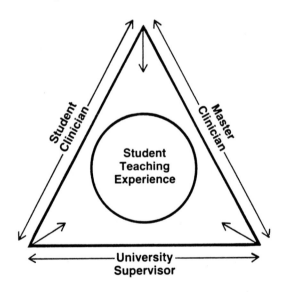

Figure 1. The student teaching TRIAD depicts *intra*dependency and *inter*dependency of the team endeavor.

University supervisors in their position as representatives of the university have a perspective of the total training program. They may have had experience in each of the TRIAD roles: that of student clinician, master clinician, and presently as university supervisor; therefore, they have a comprehensive view of what is required to complete successfully this part of the training experience.

Master clinicians bring their experiences as public school speech-language pathologists to this assignment along with the remembrance of once having been a student clinician; therefore, they are experienced in two facets of the TRIAD. It is the master clinician who has current first-hand knowledge of the school environment as a work setting. The master clinician is there to give guidance in molding an inexperienced clinician into a qualified associate whose clinical judgment and therapy skills will contribute to the success of the remedial speech and language program.

Student clinicians bring academic background and basic clinical skills to this training experience. Successful student clinicians also bring a receptive attitude to the assignment with an eagerness to assimilate experiences and suggestions. As students progress through the student teaching assignment, they will find their responsibilities for the case load a positive reinforcement toward becoming qualified speech-language pathologists.

PART I
THE STUDENT

OVERVIEW:
SIDE ONE OF THE TRIAD

Part I of this text introduces the student member of the TRIAD to speech-language-hearing services in the school setting. Part I addresses itself to three major areas: observation in the schools, student teaching in elementary schools, and student teaching at secondary sites.

Students-in-training often enter the speech-language pathology major with uncertainties about the role and responsibilities of school speech-language pathologists. Advisement periods and discussions with university faculty may give inexperienced students a partial picture of this work setting; however, a more complete understanding of the role of the speech-language pathologist in the schools comes through structured exposure to that environment.

Chapter 2 is an introduction to the school setting through observation. Basic knowledge of most school programs comes from observing speech-language pathologists in their own setting, the schools. Through observations, students become acquainted with an environment in which they may choose to work in the future. They will see the uniqueness of the schools and will be better able to decide if this is a setting that they will find rewarding and challenging. For many students-in-training, it is the first time they have returned to the schools since they completed their twelve years of compulsory education. Students-in-training who are considering this environment as a career placement have a special reason to visit the schools. It enables them to see pupils with the types of speech, language, and hearing disorders that have been discussed in the university classroom and to watch experienced speech-language pathologists practicing in school environments. This chapter discusses the purpose of observations and the role of the observer with emphasis on guidelines for being a considerate observer.

Chapter 3 defines the role and responsibilities of student clinicians in preparing for and being in the school environment. The student teaching assignment is a demanding one, and students-in-training should be aware of the expectations that will be placed upon them as well as the rewards that come from completing a task well done.

The purpose of Chapter 3 is to give student clinicians *practical* information with ideas and suggestions on how they can be successful in the school environment. Guidelines are given for performing effectively as student clinicians with a section showing how to move from dependency to independency during the school assignment. This text does not include specific remediation techniques for working with children at the elementary level, since there are texts and other publications that discuss in detail remediation techniques. Chapter 3 discusses preparation for the assignment, desirable professional qualifications, establishment of successful relationships with master clinicians and school personnel, and implementation procedures student clinicians will find invaluable as they carry out their student teaching assignments.

Chapter 4 discusses working with the adolescent who has a communication problem. A secondary assignment is an opportunity to work with pupils who are developing their self-concepts. Student clinicians who have recently been through the self-discovery process may find it stimulating to work with pupils during the turbulent years of adolescence. Working with adolescents can be challenging, rewarding, and exciting. Many students-in-training are reluctant to elect an assignment with this age group because they feel unprepared since most speech-language clinics focus primarily on the younger child. This chapter gives student clinicians basic information on how to work successfully with adolescents and tells them how to participate in a remedial program that is beneficial for pupils and student clinicians.

There has been little published material for this age level, and student clinicians will find the information and techniques described of value to them. Chapter 4 discusses developing therapeutic relationships with adolescents, logistics for operating a program in the secondary schools, and procedures and materials appropriate for adolescents.

Chapter 2

THE STUDENT OBSERVER
IN THE SCHOOL SETTING

PURPOSE OF OBSERVATIONS

Beginning Students

Observations are usually the first direct contact a beginning student has with an individual manifesting a speech-language disorder. Speech-language programs include in their curriculum a number of required observations before students assume responsibility for assessing and remediating speech-language-hearing handicapped individuals. Observations of clinical practicum have been an integral part of training programs for many years. In some training programs observations are required not only in the beginning for inexperienced students but also throughout the total training period.

The purpose of observations is twofold: (1) to enable students to see children and adults with the types of speech and language disorders that have been discussed in the university classroom and (2) to enable students to see experienced speech-language pathologists practicing in various professional settings.

At the introductory level of training, students learn about the characteristics associated with speech and language disorders. In classroom lectures, facts regarding etiology, symptoms, and characteristics of speech-language disorders are emphasized. Observations serve the purpose of taking the first step toward relating these theoretical concepts and applying them to *individuals*. After developing basic academic sophistication, students move from theoretical to applied experiences. Students have an intellectual understanding of speech-language disorders; however, textbook descriptions do not prepare them for the actual sensation of hearing disordered speech. The printed word cannot convey the sounds

11

of acoustic signals; they must be heard to be meaningful. It is necessary to move from textbook descriptions to auditory and visual realities by being with an individual manifesting these disorders.

How does an individual with nasal emission sound?

How does an individual with secondary stuttering characteristics sound?

How does a child with a lateral lisp sound?

How does a dysarthric child sound?

It is through the observation experience that students find answers to these questions. They *hear* the glottal stops, nasal snorts, and pharyngeal fricatives of the cleft palate child and *see* accompanying facial grimaces used as compensatory movements to aid in achieving acceptable acoustic quality. Students may have been exposed to the Van Riper categories of primary and secondary stuttering, and during an observation of a stuttering adolescent, the student may see behaviors that interfere with communication, such as eye blink, muscle tension, and a disturbed breathing pattern. The student will hear the slushy quality and may notice unusual facial movements of the child with a lateral lisp. Or, the student will observe the dysarthric child as he displays slurred speech, is unable to point his tongue in precise repetitive movements, and consistently misarticulates tongue tip sounds.

In the classroom typical textbook cases are studied by disorder and stereotypes for various handicapping conditions. In textbooks, cases are presented by categories, such as, laryngectomy, Down's syndrome, or cleft palate. The average case is either rare or mythical. It is a composite representation of many persons and does not allow for the range of individual differences that exist in reality. Textbook descriptions concentrate on commonalities associated with a specific disorder. During observations students hear and see that most individuals with speech-language disorders do not fit a typical textbook stereotype.

Observations give students an opportunity to see a *person* with a handicapping condition, not a *disorder* that incidentally has a human form. These cases are not disorders but *real people* with personalities, with physical appearances unique to themselves, with families, and with involvements in business, social, or school activities. They are first of all men, women, or children who have a speech-language disorder that they are attempting to remediate. Students may see a fifty-six-year-old male, an engineer, who is married, has three children and two grandchildren, is past president of Kiwanis, was formerly active in P.T.A., is well liked by business associates, and enjoys sports, traveling, and other social activities. This is a unique person who has undergone a laryngectomy and is trying to communicate with family, friends, and business associates. Or, students may observe an eight-year-old girl with a winning personality, a twelve-year-old brother who adores her, a father who is an electrician, grandparents who dote on her, a mother who is a community worker, and a family dog constantly by her side. She is training and competing in athletic events (for the handicapped), attending school (in a special education class), and learning to achieve at her optimum potential. She is a child with a handicapping condition, Down's syndrome. Another example, the label cleft palate does not give the three-dimensional picture of a person with this disorder: a little girl with pretty brown eyes, pigtails, and an infectious giggle.

Through observations, students begin to see all of these people as individuals. Classroom content must, of necessity, stress theoretical and factual information relating to the disorders. However, there is no substitute for the learning experience provided beginning students by observing individuals with speech-language disorders.

During observations, students will see experienced speech-language pathologists in various professional settings. It is here students see in practice what they have been studying in class. The student will observe that the speech-language pathologist is the dominant force in developing an environment and relationship with clients that are conducive to remediating speech-language disorders. Students will see how the speech-language pathologist structures the session for the client to obtain maximum benefit. Students will become knowledgeable of the methods employed by experienced speech-language pathologists in shaping the behavior of the client to elicit desired responses. Students will see how a competent professional develops and maintains motivation. The foregoing are important in successful therapy sessions, but achieving these are dependent upon the personal relationship established by the speech-language pathologist with a client. A good working relationship grows when an atmosphere of warmth, acceptance, and caring has been established.

During the course of several observations, students will note the diversity of personalities among speech-language pathologists and see how they achieve their basic goals. It is not the personality of the speech-language pathologist itself but the relationship established with the client that enables the competent professional to be effective.

Students will observe experienced speech-language pathologists using various techniques, which have been demonstrated in class, and will see clients responding to these techniques. Students will see a diversity of materials used in therapy and those appropriate for various clients.

Another benefit gained from observations is the opportunity to visit a variety of professional settings — public schools, hospitals, community clinics, and so forth. Many beginning students do not have a broad understanding of the diversity of professional settings in which speech-language pathologists are employed. As students gain exposure and knowledge of various work environments, they will establish a base for selecting their future professional setting.

Advanced Students

Observations enrich the professional competence of advanced students who have completed some clinical practicum. Observations become more meaningful as students acquire additional academic and clinical experiences. The student who has completed 100, 200, or more clinical hours not only is becoming a competent clinician but also is becoming a sophisticated observer. Scheduled observations throughout the training program give students information from various perspectives. At various levels of training, students are advancing in their professional competence and are able to focus attention on different components of the sessions observed. For example, a beginning student may be seeing only the basics of the therapy session, while the advanced student should be aware of the more subtle aspects of the therapeutic process. The student with some degree of sophistication has developed a sense of focus and is more alert to identifying behaviors exhibited by the clients.

Conscientious student clinicians who desire to improve their skills are aware of the areas where they need additional information, and they will attempt to select observations to fulfill their needs and interests. They may wish to observe the methods an experienced professional uses with an individual with a specific type of disorder, or they may wish to see how an on-site speech-language pathologist employs group dynamics. Observations may reinforce for students that their clinical approach is similar to those employed by experienced speech-language pathologists, thus giving a sense of confidence and security to the novice clinician. If the speech-language pathologist exhibits problems in coping with a difficult case, the novice clinician learns that easy answers are not always available, and even experienced professionals have sessions that do not run smoothly. New techniques, approaches, and methods are learned from observations.

The serious, inquiring student employs many modes for successful learning—listening and questioning (classroom lectures), watching (observations), and doing (clinical practicum). Each is part of the overall training. Each component is relevant and contributes to the competence of a qualified speech-language pathologist.

ROLE OF THE OBSERVER

A student who assumes the role of observer of a therapy session takes on many responsibilities. The main focus of this section relates to the public school setting; however, much of the discussion is relevant to other professional environments.

University Policy

Each training program establishes basic policies regarding observations. It is incumbent upon students to be knowledgeable of these policies and to follow them carefully. Observation sites are made available because faculty have made arrangements that are mutually acceptable to both the training institution and the observation site. Deviations from the mutually agreed upon conditions may jeopardize use of the facility in the future. Students may unwittingly cause problems that could impair established relationships between university and professional facilities. In one case, students were told specifically not to make contact with a particular school district. One student, however, ignored the instructions and appeared on-site without prior contact. Unfortunately, this student not only disregarded the directive that this site was not available for observations but added to the problem by being demanding, aggressive, and generally inconsiderate. The director of the district program contacted the training institution to register a sharp complaint, demanded an explanation, and suggested that if such a situation were repeated, students would no longer be given clinical experiences in that district. Considerable faculty time and effort were expended in resolving the situation. Faculty are aware that students may not realize the implications of their actions; however, students are expected to be sufficiently mature to follow established university policies.

Choosing Observation Sites

Most university programs have several observation sites available from which students may make choices. The conscientious student gives careful consideration to obtaining the best experiences. Beginning students profit from seeing a diversity of clients, settings, and personnel. More experienced students will look for observations that enrich their academic and clinical experiences. Areas that have been identified as weak, such as group dynamics and behavior management, can be strengthened by observing on-site professionals demonstrating these techniques.

Guidelines for the Considerate Observer

Student observers should have three objectives: (1) to present themselves as future professional colleagues, (2) to be good representatives of the training program, and (3) to exhibit professional and considerate conduct.

In addressing the preceding objectives, it is important that students present themselves in a manner which denotes professionalism and consideration. Following are guidelines for the considerate observer:

1. *You Are a Guest.* As an observer you have not been invited personally to the site; your presence is that of a self-invited guest. You are welcome because of arrangements made in your behalf by others; therefore, the first and foremost rule is that you conduct yourself in a professional manner at all times. Present opportunities for observations are based upon the conduct of former students, and you should assume professional responsibility to insure that your actions will enable future students to enjoy similar observational privileges.

2. *Know Why You Are Making the Observation.* You should have a clear understanding of the purpose of the observation and communicate this information to the on-site speech-language pathologist. This aids the speech-language pathologist in planning the observation so that you, the student observer, can fulfill the requirements of your assignment.

3. *Schedule Observations in Advance.* You should be prepared for no-shows. Clients may be absent on the day of your scheduled observation, and it may be necessary to reschedule your visit. If you do not plan for this contingency, you may find yourself in the unfortunate position of not being able to complete your assignment. Avoid last minute contacts. They make you look disorganized, discourteous, and uncaring, as though you were attaching little importance to the assignment. It may put the on-site speech-language pathologist in the awkward position of trying to meet your needs when it is not convenient to have a visitor.

4. *Obtain Basic Information in Advance.* When you make the initial contact, find out the hour you are to be on-site and where you are to meet the speech-language pathologist. Ask if you are to check in at the office before going to the therapy room. Inform the speech-language pathologist how long your visit is to be so that appropriate arrangements can be made. You should know if there are problems finding the entrance or if there are parking restrictions. One student parked in a convenient empty

space, which she later learned was the principal's reserved parking spot. Needless to say, that student did not make a favorable impression. If possible, plan your travel route yourself. It will save the time of persons who otherwise must give you directions.

5. *Be Flexible with Your Schedule.* As a courtesy, plan to stay for the prearranged time only. If you are invited to stay longer to see an interesting case or if the speech-language pathologist indicates there will be time later to talk with you, you may wish to remain for longer than the prearranged time. Do not leave early, as this may be interpreted to mean you did not find the experience worth your time. If it is necessary for you to leave during the middle of a session, do so as unobtrusively as possible.

6. *Be Punctual.* Being late is discourteous. Tardiness may upset the speech-language pathologist's schedule and cause undue distractions in the session. Punctuality is professional responsibility. Plan extra time for your trip; you may get lost enroute, traffic may be heavier than anticipated, or there may be difficulty in finding parking or the entrance. Plan for unexpected problems so that you will not start your observation feeling anxious and needing to apologize.

7. *Go to the Observation Alone.* Do not suggest that another student accompany you unless this has been prearranged with the on-site speech-language pathologist. The therapy room may not conveniently accommodate more than one observer, and sometimes pupils cannot tolerate the additional person. One visitor may be distracting to some children, and more may cause them to become upset.

8. *Avoid Distracting Mannerisms.* Under the best of circumstances your arrival and presence will be distracting to the pupils. Try to be as inconspicuous as possible as you find a seat, take notes, and so on. Distractions, such as a scratchy pen, turning papers, and shuffling feet, may be disturbing to others.

9. *Look Alert.* You have the responsibility to be attentive, be responsive, and learn from the situation. Nothing is more disconcerting to a professional than to have a visitor who looks bored, yawns, squirms, and acts disinterested. One stu-

dent left an unfavorable impression by looking through therapy materials while sessions were in progress. Remember, you are being viewed as a future professional colleague.

10. *Accept the Role Assigned You.* Take your cue from the speech-language pathologist regarding your involvement in the session. You may be introduced to the children, you may be invited to comment or participate in some way, or you may be virtually ignored during the therapy session. Your ability to accept the role assigned to you is a reflection of your maturity and adaptability to the situation.

11. *Plan Specific Questions to Ask.* Time is valuable, and you should use it to the best advantage by having questions prepared in advance. If the speech-language pathologist does not have time to answer your questions, you should be a gracious guest who is understanding and appreciative of the services rendered.

12. *Be Well Groomed.* Appropriate dress is expected of students. Attire worn in lecture courses may not be appropriate for professional settings. Many facilities have established dress codes in accordance with the professional image they are presenting. The well-groomed student will be welcome in any professional setting, whereas the poorly groomed observer may become an unwanted guest before the observation begins.

13. *Express Your Appreciation.* An expression of appreciation to the speech-language pathologist for the opportunity to observe is recommended. This personal acknowledgment of time and effort spent in your behalf will be appreciated. If you are unable to say thank you before leaving, a written note will convey your feeling of appreciation for the service rendered you and the university. The thoughtful student observer will personalize comments, such as, "I'm impressed with the way you worked with John," or "I like the way you have arranged your therapy space." Sharing a copy of a favorable report allows the speech-language pathologist to receive feedback of the practicum through the eyes of the observer.

14. *Notify If Unable to Keep Appointment.* If you must cancel an observation, notify the speech-language pathologist as soon as you know you are unable to attend. Sometimes special arrangements have been made for your visit, and the speech-

language pathologist must inform others of the change.

The preceding guidelines are given to create a sense of direction for being a successful observer. They are not intended to be inclusive of all the precepts of good manners and conduct. The considerate student will expand this list to include areas not specifically discussed in this section.

HOW *NOT* TO BE INVITED BACK

Following is a list of behaviors certain to make a lasting impression on any on-site speech-language pathologist:

1. Call late at night to set up urgent request for next day.
2. Establish your own procedure for making appointments.
3. Arrive late and upset speech-language pathologist's schedule.
4. Complain about the amount of work required by the university.
5. Interrupt therapy session with questions and comments.
6. Talk about pupils in front of them; after all, they really don't understand.
7. Act bored, yawn, shuffle feet, squirm in chair.
8. Read book or papers while therapy is in session.
9. Chew gum; either regular or bubble gum will do.
10. Ask if you can smoke.
11. Wear inappropriate dress and be poorly groomed.
12. Criticize what the speech-language pathologist is doing, for example, "Why are you doing . . . ?" "I've never heard of . . ." "My professor says . . ."
13. Show disappointment with types of cases seen, ages of pupils, etc.
14. Let speech-language pathologist know you have been to other observations, which were more rewarding than the present one.
15. Fail to thank the speech-language pathologist for the service rendered.
16. Be rude to office staff; you didn't come to observe them.
17. If invited to faculty room, eat heartily and don't offer to pay.

18. Let the speech-language pathologist know that "it is your day" and you should be number one. The pupils, after all, are seen frequently, but this may be the only day you will be on site. If you are successful in achieving the foregoing, you can be assured it will be the *only* time you will be on site.

Fulfilling one or more of the preceding will make you *persona non grata* at any site. This list is not meant to be all-inclusive. Creative students can devise other behaviors to add to the list.

CONCLUSION

Observations show students how their training is preparing them to become competent speech-language pathologists. Students see the application of the theoretical concepts they have learned in university training programs. Observations permit students to be in the actual setting where clients are receiving therapy for communication disorders and speech-language pathologists are functioning as professionals. The time and effort of many people have been expended in providing the experience; therefore, the greatest benefit possible should be derived from it. In preparation, students should carefully think through what the purpose of the observation is and what they hope to gain from the experience. Being well prepared makes it more meaningful. Following an observation, students should be better prepared to look beyond the textbook and relate what they are learning in the university classroom to what they have observed in the field.

Chapter 3

CLINICAL PRACTICE IN THE SCHOOLS

Each participating member of the student teaching TRIAD, student clinician, master clinician, and university supervisor, must assume basic responsibilities for the experience to be successful. This chapter will focus on the qualifications and responsibilities of the student member of the TRIAD. What follows is a guide and is not intended to be all-inclusive.

When the student teaching assignment has been made and accepted, the student should make it the *number one* priority for this period of time. The student must realize this is a demanding assignment that will require time, energy, and stamina. Attending classes can be considered a semipassive state for students inasmuch as they are the recipients of the work and effort of the university instructor. In contrast, student teaching requires active involvement of students in the practicum phase of their training; they are the doers, responsible for planning and implementing clinical procedures. In addition, they are participating in related endeavors, such as finding materials, learning about the pupils in the case load, and arranging time to confer with the master clinician and other school personnel. Student teaching is a transition period from student status to employed professional.

QUALIFICATIONS FOR ADMITTANCE TO STUDENT TEACHING

Professional Qualifications

Eligibility for a student teaching assignment requires the student to have completed a specified course of study, which includes both academic and on-campus clinical experiences. The student must realize that completion of a specified course of training is not sufficient to guarantee a successful experience in the schools. The *level of competence* that students have exhibited in their training will be a major factor in determining success in another setting. There is a basic core of knowledge and experience expected before students are assigned. Students should have demonstrated academic proficiency in several areas:

1. Knowledge of psychological, physical, emotional, social, and cognitive aspects of growth and development
2. Knowledge of etiologies, characteristics, and manifestations associated with individuals with language, speech, and hearing disorders
3. Ability to develop, implement, and evaluate appropriate remediation procedures

Demonstrated clinical competence is a prerequisite to a student teaching assignment. It has been recommended that a minimum of 100 hours of on-campus speech, language, and hearing practicum is necessary to show competency in writing behavioral objectives, preparing lesson plans, implementing therapy, evaluating remediation procedures, report writing, and other professional activities (Monnin and Peters, 1977). On-campus clinical practicum usually includes experiences with children of various ages and disorders. It is advantageous if students have had previous experience with children as a school aide, camp counselor, or youth group adviser. Students benefit from these experiences by increasing their awareness of childhood and adolescent behaviors in various environments. Students who have had experience in working with normal children are aware of individual differences that are considered to be within the range of normality. This background enables student clinicians to evaluate more effectively the performance of an exceptional child.

Personal Qualifications

There are many personal qualities that effective clinicians possess, for example, an effective clinician is able to establish rapport with children and adults. It is not unusual for beginning clinicians to have concerns about being liked by clients, and they may be so involved with trying to please their clients that their objectivity as clinicians may be impaired. Rapport does not mean that a student must become "one of the kids." It is not possible for an adult to become the peer of a five- or ten-year-old child, and student clinicians should not attempt to do so. Children do not need or want a twenty-five- or thirty-five-year-old friend. They want friends their own age who can share with them the joys, anxieties, and special secrets only other children their age can appreciate. Children, however, do need a friendly, mature, caring adult who offers stability, understanding, and acceptance of them as they are trying to fulfill their communication potential and all that it implies. It is particularly essential for young clinicians working with secondary school pupils to maintain the client-clinician relationship; to attempt to become one of the crowd will lead to an ineffectual program. Rather than improving communication, there will be a negative response resulting in a breakdown of communication. To establish rapport is to develop and maintain an effective clinical working relationship.

Additional desirable personal qualities include professional attitude; personal integrity; ability to assume responsibility; ability to establish a leadership role; self-starter; reliability; responsiveness to constructive criticism; flexibility; ability to adapt to changing situations; maturity; ethical behavior; responsive to needs of others; a caring, understanding, and accepting nature; and a sense of humor. A sense of humor enables student clinicians to maintain their equilibrium in trying times and also makes them more approachable by pupils and school personnel. Student clinicians are encouraged to assess these personal qualities within themselves and to assume responsibility for evaluating their strengths and weaknesses in these areas.

First impressions frequently are the most important, and they are based on the image one projects. Appearance and grooming play a major role in how one is perceived by others. Student clinicians should choose wearing apparel that is clean, neat, and appropriate for the school site. Selecting fabrics that are durable, hold a press, and are attractive in color are considerations. Student clinicians should avoid clothing and jewelry that are fussy and cause distractions, such as heavy bracelets that jangle or rings that catch on stockings and sweaters. Major factors contributing to a well-groomed appearance are cleanliness, good posture, and hairstyles that allow the face to be seen. A general feeling of vitality is an important quality a student clinician wants to project. Student clinicians should be aware that poor posture often portrays one as being ineffectual, tired, and timid.

Books have been written on body language, and most students will have some awareness of stances and postures that reveal attitudes through unspoken language. There are cultural differences that exist in body messages, and student clinicians may wish to learn more about nonverbal communication through readings, courses, or discussions.

PURPOSE OF BEING A STUDENT CLINICIAN

The student teaching experience introduces students to the practical application of clinical speech and language in public education. Throughout the assignment they are gaining exposure and developing skills appropriate for this work environment. Participating with an experienced school speech-language pathologist enables students to grow from novice clinician to associate clinician status.

The school setting is unique insofar as it provides experiences not available in any other environment. In no other setting are children housed in an organized program for so many hours a day and for so many months in a year. The clinician has the opportunity to assess large numbers of children, observe children in a nontherapeutic environment, peruse children's school records, contact school personnel, and observe children in a peer group environment.

Students have an opportunity to learn how school speech-language programs are organized. Effective planning is necessary in order to incorporate all the activities that must be accomplished during the school day. As student clinicians learn to organize a clinical program, they will find they must schedule time for therapy, referrals, testing, record keeping, and contacts with teachers and other school personnel, as well as conferences with parents.

Student teaching is an opportunity for students to improve and strengthen their competency in an actual work environment. Employers are interested in hiring competent speech-language pathologists, and careful consideration is given to applicants' performance in the environment for which they are seeking employment. Student teaching long has been recognized as an invaluable part of the training of qualified speech-language pathologists for the schools. It is for this reason that state departments of education require on-site experience before public school certification is awarded.

PREPARING FOR THE ASSIGNMENT

Student responsibilities prior to applying for a student teaching assignment include (1) being knowledgeable of university requirements for student teaching, (2) meeting all prerequisites, (3) meeting established deadlines for application for a student teaching assignment, (4) knowing state requirements for certification, and (5) knowing procedures for obtaining state certification.

It is helpful when students provide master clinicians and university supervisors with an education and work experience résumé. Résumés are most useful when they include educational background, clinical experiences including types of cases seen, previous work experiences, particularly those involving contact with children, and special interests in assignments, such as working with hearing impaired, multiply handicapped, or developmentally disabled children. Résumés have aided master clinicians and university supervisors in planning practical school experiences for student clinicians.

Mature students will anticipate the demands of the assignment. They will plan in advance of the assignment how they will meet transportation needs. For most students this will mean an automobile in good dependable running condition. Financial situations must be considered. Some students will need to make arrangements for loans or arrange for part-time jobs. Students who must work while in student teaching should plan well in advance so that their work schedules will not conflict with the assignment. It may be said that short of divorce or abandonment, family commitments must not interfere with the student teaching schedule or performance. Students will have varying family commitments, and they must find the best means for handling their particular situation. (This is not the time to plan a big wedding or give birth to triplets.) A frank discussion with the university supervisor may be helpful in problem solving areas of concern to the student. The old adage "Two heads are better than one" may apply here.

Master clinicians have expressed concern about students allowing themselves sufficient time to participate fully in the opportunities available during the student teaching experience, such as participating in media centers, faculty meetings, and in-service training (*Conference on Standards for Supervised Experience for Speech and Hearing Specialists in Public Schools,* 1969). Program requirements vary from training institution to training institution, but students must be realistic about the additional course work they will undertake; they must be cautious and not overcommit themselves.

BEGINNING THE ASSIGNMENT

Relationship with Master Clinician

Establishing an effective working relationship with the master clinician is of prime importance. Master clinicians are chosen because they are willing to participate in the training program; they are eager to share their expertise and try to make the initial impact of the assignment as nonthreatening as possible.

Helpful suggestions in establishing a good relationship:

1. Be responsive to the master clinician's sharing of introductory information.
2. Be receptive to the master clinician's opinions, point of view, and method of conducting therapy.
3. Show respect for those activities the master clinician is performing to fulfill the work assignment.
4. Be prepared for the assignment so that anxiety can be managed without pressure being placed on the master clinician.

Sometimes students focus only on clinical performance and fail to realize the importance of other behaviors necessary for satisfactory professional relationships. *Word to the wise:* (1) be punctual, (2) be reliable in commitments, (3) be neatly groomed, (4) be prepared, (5) do not prejudge master clinicians and their mode of operating, and (6) reserve judgment about information provided by other students.

Students must be cognizant that the master clinician's first responsibility is to the pupils served. In the academic environronment students are the main concern of the faculty; however, master clinicians are held accountable for the progress of the pupils in their schools. Student clinicians must adapt to a situation in which they are not the first responsibility of the master clinician. The school program was established not to train university students but to remediate pupils. Master clinicians have assumed an added function by their willingness to become involved in the university training program.

Relationship with Pupils

The successful clinician establishes appropriate clinical relationships with pupils. Most student clinicians have had previous speech-language clinical experience with young children, and the skills acquired in developing clinical relationships with these children can be transferred to the school environment. Some students may have had prior experiences with groups of children, and some have not had any such experiences. If students have not worked with groups of children, it is their responsibility to seek information regarding group dynamics and managing group behavior.

Student clinicians must learn to cope with what often seems to be an unending stream of children arriving for therapy. It is necessary for the student clinician to become adept at bidding farewell to one group of children while simultaneously welcoming the next group of eager youngsters. Often there is no break time between therapy sessions, and student clinicians must be prepared to move with ease and promptness into the next session. Advance planning and organization are required to avoid a delay in beginning therapy, which not only wastes valuable time but also may result in losing the attention of the children. It is incumbent upon the student clinician to utilize efficiently and effectively the limited time that is available to each child in the case load.

One of the most difficult areas for the novice student clinician is dealing effectively with the high school age pupil. If a student clinician has an assignment at the secondary level, additional time and attention is required to develop skill in working with this age pupil. Speech-language programs for the adolescent are discussed in Chapter 4.

Meeting Program Requirements

Students should be knowledgeable of university program requirements for the student teaching assignment. If there are instances when not all requirements can be met at an assigned site, the student should discuss the situation with the master clinician, who may have suggestions for alternative methods for meeting the requirements. The master clinician may be able to use contacts in the school district for some requirements to be met at a different site. If the master clinician is unable to provide the necessary experiences, it is the responsibility of the student to inform the university supervisor. Then the student and university supervisor can plan together how these requirements will be met.

DURING THE ASSIGNMENT

Students should be aware they have specific responsibilities during the student teaching assignment. Frequently they are not cognizant of these personal and professional obligations. When asked, "What is your responsibility as a student clinician?" they often reply, "To do what we are told to do." Obviously, success in the assignment transcends this response. Master clinicians and university supervisors are guides, but students must realize they are accountable for their own learning and professional behaviors.

The following discussion encompasses both personal and professional qualities that master clinicians and university supervisors have reported are necessary for a successful student teaching experience.

Communicating with Master Clinician
and University Supervisor

The foundation for a successful working relationship is laid when the student shares in the responsibility of establishing open communication with the master clinician. An attitude of mutual trust and cooperation is founded upon an open exchange of information. Once a meaningful dialogue has been established, it is possible for student clinician and master clinician to discuss freely areas of importance to the student. Master clinicians' experience in the schools enables them to give input to student clinicians regarding their role as emerging independent clinicians. A reflective response to master clinicians' input helps students mature into competent professionals. Learning to assess one's strengths and weaknesses is an ongoing but difficult process; however, sharing with perceptive master clinicians helps student clinicians realize more fully their own potential. Sometimes, because of anxiety, student clinicians are too insecure to communicate freely with their master clinicians, thus isolating themselves from a ready source of help. It is unfortunate if student clinicians do not avail themselves of the opportunity to communicate with their master clinicians.

The university supervisor also is interested in the student's success in the school assignment. Knowing the effort students expend to become eligible for student teaching, the university supervisor desires this to be a successful endeavor. The competent student clinician is a credit to the university program and a source of satisfaction to the university supervisor. Students will find most supervisors willing to counsel them when they come for advice. Often the supervisor's experience helps student clinicians to comprehend better the student teaching assignment as it relates to the broad horizons of the field of speech-language pathology.

Student clinicians may find they need to schedule conferences with their university supervisor in regard to the requirements of the assignment. They should inform their supervisor if required student teaching experiences cannot be provided at the assigned school location. When appropriate, university supervisors will arrange for these experiences to be acquired at another site.

Expectations of the master clinician may not always be realistic. The demands may be either too stringent or not sufficiently challenging. Talking through this situation with the university supervisor may enable the student to understand what is realistic and aid the student in discussing these concerns with the master clinician.

Generally a good working relationship, even a friendly one, develops between student clinician and master clinician. There are, however, instances when a personality conflict may arise, which makes a good learning experience difficult to achieve. The student clinician should feel free to discuss this with the university supervisor. The university supervisor is in a position to make valuable suggestions or take appropriate action.

Interpersonal Relationships

The success of the speech-language program is proportionate to the support it receives from school personnel; therefore, to work effectively in the school environment, it is necessary to establish good rapport with all school personnel. Classroom teachers and others can provide invaluable assistance to pupils receiving therapy. One of the opportunities provided during student teaching is learning to relate effectively with allied personnel. A district personnel director has stated, "Many teachers fail because of their inability to work cooperatively in the school setting" (Gage, 1979). The facility to establish rapport with others is an elusive quality, which may be described as exhibiting tact, diplomacy, empathy, and willingness to be part of a team effort. Most people form opinions based on personal observations. School personnel generally do not have the background to judge the clinical competence of the speech-language pathologist; therefore, they frequently evaluate the merit of the speech and language program on their perception of the personal qualities of the individual speech-language pathologist.

Dependability

Dependability is the basis for building a trusting relationship. To be dependable is to demonstrate commitment to a goal. Within this framework are such characteristics as (1) being punctual, (2) meeting commitments, (3) being prepared with lesson plans and materials, (4) adhering to a daily schedule, (5) picking up and returning children to their classrooms at designated times, (6) using time wisely, (7) using and returning materials promptly, and (8) notifying appropriate personnel when unable to keep commitments.

Accepting Constructive Criticism

Students should seek ways to change behaviors that are not compatible with the assignment. Students' abilities to use criticism as a foundation for change enables them to develop greater potential. Although few students wish to hear negative comments, a positive attitude toward constructive criticism is an aid to the successful completion of a student teaching assignment. Defensive behaviors such as denial, excuses, rationalization, and intellectualization are self-defeating for a student clinician. Willingness to accept constructive criticism enables student clinicians to benefit from comments and suggestions given by master clinicians and university supervisors.

Resourcefulness: Problem Solving

During the school day unexpected events arise that are beyond the control of student clinicians. Situations occur that are beyond the control of master clinicians, too! To be resourceful is to problem solve, to find an alternate solution when indicated, and to think on your feet. It behooves students to develop skills for meeting unforseen occurrences and learn to be resourceful in developing contingency plans. Resourcefulness encompasses the elusive quality of *creativity*, which implies imagination, innovation, originality, and uniqueness. Students who demonstrate these qualities are flexible and capable of adjusting to changing situations.

For the professional eager to do a competent job, logistical breakdown is frustrating and disheartening. It is the little things that go wrong which may cause a devoted professional to resort to ineffectual practices. Areas in which problems may occur and often do are the following:

1. Getting the children to therapy — and on time.
2. Getting notations written before the next group of children arrives.
3. Having materials ready for the next group.
4. Coping with last minute changes in school schedules.
5. Getting information to teachers.

The astute student clinician will have developed contingency plans for the little things that go wrong or need special attention in the daily schedule. Having successfully resolved minor logistical problems, the resourceful student clinician is in a position to meet and cope with major crises when, and if, they occur.

How resourceful would you be if the following incident were to arise?

Situation: Knowing your university supervisor is coming to observe, you have prepared carefully your best therapy plans. You arrive on-site laden with materials and backup techniques to insure an outstanding performance. You alerted your kids last week, and they know your supervisor is coming to *evaluate you.*

Problem: The school secretary meets you with a smile and informs you that half the children are absent with chicken pox. Your morning groups are in this category.

Solution: Look over your available options.

1. Can you bring the afternoon pupils in for therapy?
2. Can you do a diagnostic evaluation?
3. Can you find a pupil on carry-over and bring him in for therapy and reassessment?
4. Can you introduce the university supervisor, who raises rottweilers, to the principal, who breeds rottweilers?
5. Can you come up with a super solution of your own that will satisfy all requirements?

Learning to cope with such occurrences tries the soul of the most seasoned professional, but for the emerging professional, these events can be traumatic. By using resourcefulness and a sense of humor to solve the predicament, the student clinician may find a way to resolve the situation to everyone's satisfaction.

Maturity and Self-Reliance

Mature student clinicians are self-directed. They are capable of taking direction and operating as part of a team effort, but they do not wait to be told what to do and how to function. They show independence, initiative, and self-reliance. Established requirements of the assignment are the baseline from which they operate. Mature self-directed students are not content with fulfilling the minimum requirements; they are constantly seeking ways to add to their experiences.

Dependent/Independent

At the beginning of the student teaching assignment, it is expected the student clinician will be dependent upon the master clinician for direction. As students become familiar with the environment and gain confidence, they should begin to move away from being dependent in their professional behavior, interpersonal relationships, and clinical practicum. Semidependence is that middle ground where student clinicians are no longer completely dependent on the master clinician for all decisions, but they are not yet sufficiently experienced to assume full responsibility for the program. Independence is achieved when the student clinician is ready to leave the supervised environment to function independently as a professional. Figure 2 shows how a student clinician may be expected to move from a state of being dependent to becoming independent in the assignment.

Growth

Lack of continuing adequate growth is tantamount to regression. Growth is shown by making consistent progress throughout the student teaching assignment. What may be acceptable performance in the early stages of training is not necessarily considered satisfactory for the more experienced student clinician. Growth is achieved by evaluating the present level of performance and working toward effecting modifications that lead to personal and professional maturity.

Growth in and of itself is not necessarily sufficient to indicate clinical competence. For example, on a rating scale of 1 to 7, student A starts at point 1 and progresses to point 4, while student B starts at point 3 and progresses to point 6. Both students improved by three points; however, their clinical performance would not be judged equal. Although growth is important and indicative of future professional achievement, the final level of competence attained is the factor by which professional performance is measured.

Ability to Generalize

The ability to generalize is a major factor in achieving competency as a clinician. The student who has the ability to generalize is capable of reasoning inductively, synthesizing information, and expanding from the specific to the whole. Such a student is able to make the relationship between past and present and theorize toward the future. Although student teaching is a new experience, the alert student takes information from past personal and professional experiences and applies it to new situations. The competent student is able to project the essential components to form the gestalt.

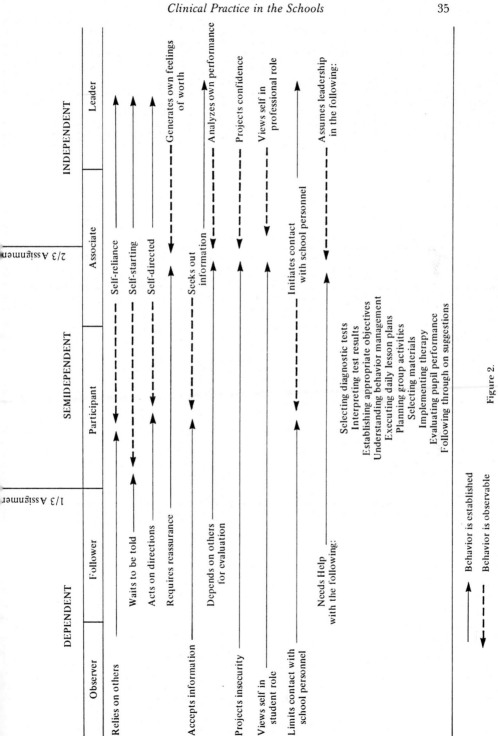

Figure 2.

Expressive Skills

Those who enter the profession of speech-language pathology tend to be verbal and articulate. Student clinicians are expected to have assessed carefully their own speech, language, and vocal patterns since, in any setting, they will be the models for those seeking remediation. The mobility of the population makes it incumbent upon clinicians to be aware of the speech and dialect spoken in the area in which they are working as well as their own regional characteristics.

The hallmark of an effective communicator is the ability to organize thoughts and make a clear, concise presentation. Speech-language pathologists frequently are asked to make presentations to school faculties, P.T.A.s, and service organizations. Most students, as part of their undergraduate general education, may have completed a course in oral communication. Students who find it difficult to make an oral presentation, either prepared or extemporaneous, benefit by taking appropriate course work or seeking opportunities to speak before an audience.

Student clinicians should be prepared to use their expressive skills to further public relations. Administrative and community support is vital to the success of any speech and language program, and the conscientious speech-language pathologist seeks ways to advertise within the school system and the community the effectiveness of the program.

Student clinicians have reported one of the most difficult tasks is to discuss a speech and language problem in terms that can be understood by those not in the field. When clinicians are asked to explain their speech and language program to school personnel, parent groups, and community organizations, they must be prepared to use vocabulary that is comprehended readily by their audience.

Another necessary ability for all clinicians is good clinical report writing, a skill that some have and some need to develop. A sign of professionalism is the ability to write reports that are comprehensible to the reader. It is important to be clear, concise, and write with a specific audience in mind: principals, classroom teachers, nurses, psychologists, and parents. Student teaching provides opportunities for report writing. For student clinicians who have difficulty with spelling or sentence structure or who feel insecure about their writing skills, it is recommended they take appropriate course work.

Ethical Practices

It is expected student clinicians will adhere to the ethical practices of their profession whenever and wherever they are conducting clinical procedures. They must remember that information they acquire about the pupils in their case load is to be treated with the utmost confidentiality. Federal and state laws are specific about rights to privacy, and student clinicians should assume responsibility for learning school policy and district implementation procedures for fulfilling their ethical responsilities.

Self-Evaluation

Ongoing self-evaluation is essential if continued professional growth is to be expected. Master clinicians and university supervisors expect student clinicians to develop the ability to evaluate their performance on both personal and professional levels. Realistic self-assessment enables student clinicians to become more objective about their performance in the schools. They should be aware of positive attributes so they may use these qualities to their best advantage, as well as being able to identify changes that are needed.

Students will find the use of videotapes helpful in evaluating their effectiveness as speech-language clinicians. The self-evaluation process includes assessment of integration of academic knowledge with clinical skills, as well as voice, grooming, posture, and body language. It is important that guidelines be established for the student clinician either by the master clinician or the university supervisor. Establishing directions and giving students points of focus enables them to perceive the value of using videotaping as a learning experience (Culatta and Helmick, 1980). With established guidelines and proper demonstration of how to view the tapes for self-evaluation, student clinicians can observe themselves and evaluate their personal and professional behaviors.

Beyond academic knowledge and clinical skills, areas of assessment include establishing good relationships with master clinicians, pupils, school personnel and university supervisors; taking responsibility and being dependable; being resourceful; demonstrating maturity and self-reliance; accepting suggestions and constructive criticism; and using expressive skills effectively. Rate yourself on each of the personal and professional qualities discussed in the chapter. First, evaluate your present level of performance by identifying areas of strengths and areas that need additional growth. Second, define and establish appropriate goals for yourself in those areas needing improvement. Plan specific ways to reach these goals and set time limits for achieving them. Third, at the specified time, reassess your level of performance and define and establish new goals. As you become more competent, your self-evaluation and goals become more sophisticated. *Remember*: Self-improvement is an ongoing process.

HOW TO BE *UNSUCCESSFUL*

The unsuccessful student clinician displays one or more of the following characteristics:

A. Manipulates others and is reticent to share information with university supervisor and master clinician. Hesitates to express self throughout the assignment because of overwhelming fear of a poor evaluation.

B. Views poor interpersonal relationships with children, peers, and supervisor as being due to unresponsiveness on the part of others.

C. Is late, unprepared, unorganized, and undependable.

D. Is inflexible; desires to change the situation to fit personal needs.

E. Assumes no personal responsibility for failure; always has an excuse for things that go wrong; does not anticipate or prepare for possible problems.

F. Employs frequent use of the following:

If only . . .	I didn't have the course . . .
I didn't know . . .	The professor was no good . . .
Nobody told me . . .	No one can expect me to . . .

It's unfair . . .   It's a personality conflict . . .

Tell me how . . .   Nobody understands my problem . . .

G. Is incapable of dealing with a problem. When difficulties arise, has no sources or resources available.

H. Uses materials and therapy techniques in the same way as initially demonstrated (noncreative).

I. Is dependent on others throughout the student teaching assignment. Requires constant direction to function:

Waits to be told,

Asks to be shown, and

Functions only under direct supervision.

J. Is satisfied with small amount of growth. Suspect the following phrases:

I need more experience.

I need more confidence.

I need more course work.

I do better when no one is observing me.

K. Views skills in oral and written communication as unimportant. Writes reports that are incomprehensible to others.

L. Never evaluates self realistically in relation to level of performance and interpersonal relationships. Resists changes in behavior to achieve appropriate personal goals. Uses phrases, such as, "This is the way I am," "I don't want to change," "It's not necessary for me to change," "It's not my problem" (see F).

M. Approaches all situations as a first experience. Two and two never add up to four. When given specific information for one situation, *avoids* expanding this basic information for use in other appropriate situations. See Figure 3.

IMPLEMENTING PROFESSIONAL SKILLS

Throughout the academic program the student has been exposed to a body of information that is to be utilized and implemented during the student teaching experience. Students are expected to show growth in their ability to integrate theoretical concepts and relate this knowledge to the practicum setting by performing competently and effectively in the areas of identification, assessment, remediation, and evaluation of language, speech, and hearing pupils. The integration of theoretical knowledge with clinical

RATING SCALE

On a five point scale:
1 equals baseline
5 equals competence

The unsuccessful student will score as follows:

Experience	*Initial Rating*		*Final Rating*
1st experience:	starts at 1.0	———➤	progresses to 2.0
2nd experience:	starts at 1.0	———➤	progresses to 2.0
3rd experience:	starts at 1.0	———➤	progresses to 2.0

TO BE MOST UNSUCCESSFUL, NEVER PROGRESS BEYOND POINT 2.0

Figure 3. The rating scale shows students how to *avoid* success in practicum assignments.

practicum is the foundation from which successful experiences are built.

Beginning Therapy

Most students are eager to start working with pupils as soon as they begin their student teaching assignment. Some students are frustrated not to be given the entire case load when they arrive on site, whereas other students are hesitant to take over the responsibility of the case load. When student clinicians begin therapy depends upon the philosophy of the master clinician. Some master clinicians are reluctant to be observed conducting therapy, fearing it will stifle the creativity of the student clinician. Other master clinicians want the student to observe for an extended period of time. It has proven most beneficial for students to observe their master clinicians for two or three sessions before becoming involved directly in the clinical activities. Students may start by working with only a few pupils and gradually increase the number until they are responsible for the entire case load.

It is not always easy for the master clinician to relinquish responsibility of the case load to the student clinician. It is important for students to remember that the master clinician is the person legally responsible for the progress of the-pupils in the case load. In addition, master clinicians may have worked with some of these children for an extended period of time, and a close personal relationship has evolved. Another factor for students to understand is that changing clinicians requires the children to make an adjustment to someone new who will be working with them for a limited period of time.

The student clinician, in consultation with the master clinician, should gradually assume total responsibility for assessment, scheduling, planning, and implementing remediation. In the actual job situation, speech-language pathologists must rely on their own resources. Usually there will not be other speech-language pathologists on site to give guidance; therefore, it is imperative that student clinicians avail themselves of the opportunity to function as independently as possible.

Group Therapy

Scheduling pupils for either individual or group therapy is based on meeting the needs of each individual pupil. A therapy group may range from two children to four or more. Some pupils are best served by receiving individual therapy, while others are more responsive when working with other pupils. If group therapy is indicated, criteria must be established for forming groups; age, types of disorder, personal qualities, and other factors should be taken into consideration when scheduling children (Neidecker, 1980).

Consultation with master clinician and university supervisor can help in establishing realistic criteria for meeting the needs of individual children in a group session. Group therapy requires skills in handling group interaction, group dynamics, and group responses (Cartwright and Zander, 1960; Backus, 1957). The student clinician must become competent in establishing individual objectives *within* the group objectives. Although establishing objectives for both the individuals and the group may seem complex, the ultimate objectives remain the same, attaining speech-language competence for each pupil.

In group therapy sessions, it is important to use peer interaction to stimulate growth in communication skills. An important function of group sessions is to develop an interdependency among pupils instead of the traditional dependency on the speech-language clinician only (Lewin, 1951). Appropriate use of *peer* interaction often can be more productive than *clinician-peer* interaction.

With peer interaction there is added stimulation in the speech-language sessions. Student clinicians should be sufficiently adept in group dynamics to avoid one child dominating the entire session or allowing another child to remain in the background and receive too little attention and practice in the group session.

Student clinicians should be knowledgeable of the benefits group sessions offer speech-language pupils:

1. There are opportunities for child-child interaction in group sessions.
2. Children often feel reassured when they know other children have similar speech-language problems.
3. There can be peer reinforcement of new behaviors in and out of therapy sessions.
4. Groups foster a more lifelike environment in which children learn to compete and cooperate.
5. Group sessions can be motivating and stimulating for both children and speech-language pathologists.
6. Some activities lend themselves to group exercises that are not possible in individual sessions.

Careful preparation is necessary when planning group therapy lessons:

1. Activities should be general enough for each child to work at his own level; children progress at different rates; even groups that start with all the children at the same level do not remain homogeneous.
2. Each child should know his own behavioral objective.
3. There is a need to promote peer encouragement, not an atmosphere of criticism.
4. Activities need to include child-child interaction; otherwise, the sessions are individual therapy with more than

one child present.

Group therapy requires skill in behavior management. Two important parts of behavior management are developing timing and pacing within speech-language sessions. *Timing* is planning the appropriate length of a session and the number of activities used within the session. *Pacing* is developing a technique that enables the sessions to proceed smoothly. It is speeding up or slowing down a session, which is accomplished by the rate of speech used by the clinician, presentation of materials during the session, expectation of the number of responses from the pupils, and so forth. It is important for student clinicians to understand the art of using a variety of pacing methods in order to provide stimulation and motivation in therapy. Momentum of the sessions has much to do with the success of the therapeutic process.

Materials

Materials should be used as a tool in learning and should not be considered of primary importance in the remediation process. The judicious use of materials will serve as a valuable aid to clinicians, but they must never be used as a substitute for clinical skills. As student clinicians move through their practicum assignments, they are developing a materials bank, which they will use when they are professionals in the field.

Student clinicians will be seeing many pupils with all types of speech and language disorders and a wider age range than they have seen previously in the campus speech-language clinic. Selecting and using appropriate materials for this diversified group is a skill in itself. It is a sign of skill and creativity when a clinician can use a limited number of materials and adapt them to a variety of effective training experiences.

In the itinerant school speech-language programs, students clinicians may find they are required to move from one setting to another in the course of a day, just as they will do when they are working as professionals in the schools. Materials that are compact, durable, and adaptable for different populations, age groups, and various speech-language disorders will best serve the clinician in conducting therapy.

The number of commercial and programmed materials is increasing as evidenced by the mailings speech-language pathologists receive from publishing firms. It seems at times as if all the world is in business to sell materials for pupils with communication disorders. It is important that students learn to evaluate and use materials effectively, and student teaching is an excellent environment for learning this.

Student clinicians need to know how to evaluate, adapt, and use materials appropriate for specialized populations, such as the severe cerebral palsied, the developmentally disabled, groups of children, and adolescents at the secondary level. There are various sources of materials for student clinicians to explore as they do their school practicum. The most available sources are master clinicians, university supervisors, and fellow students. For the innovative student clinician, found articles prove a challenge. Such materials can be from recycled sources and are "second time 'round" articles. Thrift stores, such as The Salvation Army and Goodwill, are treasure houses for some student clinicians.

Some student organizations have sponsored workshops on their campuses in which effective use of materials have been displayed and demonstrated. Creative students will invent, devise, fashion, and produce their own materials based on input from other sources.

Special Abilities

Many student clinicians overlook special skills and talents they possess, which can be incorporated into therapy sessions. Sometimes student clinicians are hesitant to use their special talents because they do not realize the significance and value of using nonconventional clinical procedures. Student clinicians should do a careful, honest self-appraisal of their strengths and talents and plan ways in which they can incorporate these skills into the therapeutic process. Conscientious student clinicians prepare appropriate and realistic short-term and long-term objectives for each pupil. Then they must determine the best methods to help their pupils achieve these objectives, i.e. drill, programmed lessons, stories, role playing, art, singing, or other creative activities. With many pupils, a direct approach is most effective; with other pupils, indirect or creative techniques may be more productive. Student clinicians may expand their clinical repertoire by introducing activities that employ their special talents, such as singing, guitar playing, and creative dramatics. *Special activities* not only help the difficult-to-motivate pupil, but also supplement regular therapy procedures and aid carry-over with other pupils. When student clinicians draw upon their special abilities and talents, they are developing their creative and artistic potential as well as providing their pupils with additional therapeutic approaches to improve their communication skills.

Use of Equipment

The availability of technical instruments for use in therapy is expanding continually. Videotaping is one valuable teaching aid that can be incorporated into the remediation process. In almost all campus speech-language clinics, students have been exposed to the advantages of using tape recorders, Language Masters®, and other valuable equipment aids. Student clinicians should be aware of computer-age instruments for the severely handicapped, such as, electronic typewriters, language boards, voice machines, other nonoral equipment for the handicapped, and newly developed instruments. The alert clinician will plan ways to use modern technology to help expedite the communication needs of their pupils.

Films

There are films that may be used as classroom or therapy room activities. Imaginative speech-language pathologists can make films meaningful for both speech-language improvement and speech-language remediation. An example is the film *Tops* (Eames). It has no narrative but can be utilized in therapy settings in a variety of ways. Many different objectives can be implemented through the use of this film, for example, articulation, sequencing activities, categorizing, vocabulary building, and body movement. Other films can also be used for many diversified objectives. Films can serve as motivation for pupils while furthering the objectives of the speech-language session.

Organizing and Compiling an Information-Material File

Throughout the student teaching assignment, students collect materials, information, and handouts from observations, conferences, in-service meetings, and workshops. Master clinicians offer students opportunities to duplicate or copy materials they find useful in therapy. Material that has been collected carefully should be organized so it can be retrieved easily when needed. It is suggested that students purchase a large portable plastic file, which is useful for organizing materials, handouts, resource information, and so forth. The materials they have collected can be divided and filed under general categories and subcategories. As an example, under the general category of articulation may be several subcategories pertaining to specific phonological disorders. Under each subcategory are materials, suggested activities, and appropriate techniques for remediation of that specific disorder.

Lesson plans and case study reports also should be kept in the file. Students will find this information useful when writing reports or seeking information on cases in the future. Retaining particularly well chosen phrases or appropriate terminology can be helpful as a reference at a later time. Having an organized information-material file is particularly beneficial during the first year of professional employment.

Interpersonal Relationships

Successful school speech-language pathologists will attest to the necessity of establishing and maintaining effective public relations. Laws can mandate, but unless the school speech-language pathologist strives to establish and maintain professional relationships and open lines of communication with others in the school environment, the speech and language program lacks a component essential for success. Social amenities are important in maintaining professional relationships. Coffee break etiquette and diplomacy are two of the many areas that contribute to maintaining a good working relationship.

As has been stated earlier, it is important for the student clinician to establish good interpersonal relationships with school personnel — administrators, teachers, office staff, aides, consultants, and health service personnel. As student clinicians move through their student teaching experience, they should avail themselves of opportunities to mingle with classroom teachers, consult with them frequently, and involve them in the program.

Classroom teachers are with the children during the major portion of the school day; therefore, enlisting the classroom teacher's aid and expertise will help children transfer what they have learned in therapy to the classroom situation. Teachers have a direct interest in the success of their pupils; so, involving them in the program elicits their support for the program. Also, any seasoned school speech-language pathologist can verify there are two people who deserve special attention—the secretary and the custodian. The tasks of many clinicians have been made lighter by the interest and cooperation of the secretary and custodian. The secretary may find some extra construction paper, and the custodian may locate additional chairs.

Relationship to Communication Aides

Many student clinicians will find communication aides on-site when they begin their assignments. If communication aides are present, university supervisors and master clinicians expect student clinicians to learn to work with these paraprofessionals. As described by Schubert, the purpose for having an aide is "to reduce the time and effort of the professional in administering minimal tasks so that the clinician can increase and intensify his efforts with the more complex communicative disordered person" (1978, p. 127). He further states that the duties are usually determined by the needs of the institution in which aides are hired; however, the communication aide always works under the direct supervision of a certified speech-language pathologist. Communication aides supplement the services of the speech-language pathologist by (1) using programmed remediation techniques with selected speech-language handicapped pupils, (2) preparing materials for pupil's use, (3) acting as an assistant in organizing activities and direction for pupils in the case load, (4) recording language samples, (5) administering and scoring tests, (6) instructing pupils in remedial techniques, (7) developing audio tapes for pupil's use, and (8) maintaining materials and files. A communication aide enables pupils to receive more intensive and frequent therapy and should not be used to increase clinical case loads.

The use of supportive personnel to provide supplemental services is not new in the field of speech-language pathology. Guidelines were established in 1970 by the American Speech and Hearing Association for the role, training, and supervision of the communication aide (ASHA, 1970). These guidelines have been updated by the American Speech-Language-Hearing Association to reflect federal legislation and language usage of the 1980s (ASHA, 1981).

In the 1981 guideline, the term suggested for supportive personnel is Speech-Language Assistant and/or Audiology Assistant. The qualifications, training, and duties of supportive personnel as described in the guidelines are as follows:

Qualification of the Speech-Language Assistant and Audiology Assistant

The following minimum qualifications should be considered in selecting individuals for employment as speech-language or audiology assistants:
1. A high school diploma or the equivalent;
2. Communication skills adequate for the tasks assigned;
3. Ability to relate to the clinical population being served.

Additional qualifications may be established according to the needs of the program and the population being served.

Training of the Speech-Language Assistant and Audiology Assistant

... emphasis should be on competency-based skill acquisition ... Training may be provided through formal course work, workshops, observation and/or supervised practicum. Methods of training shall be determined according to the needs and resources of the work setting.

Appropriate areas for training may include any or all of the following:
1. Normal processes in speech, language, and hearing;
2. Disorders of speech, language, and hearing;
3. Behavior management skills;
4. Response discrimination skills including but not limited to the discrimination of correct/incorrect verbal responses along the dimensions of speech sound production, voice parameters, fluency, syntax and semantics;
5. Program administration skills including stimulus presentation and consequation, data collection and reporting procedures and utilization of programmed instructional materials;

6. Equipment and materials used in the assessment and/or management of speech, language, and hearing disorders;

7. Overview of professional ethics and their application to the assistant's activities. (p. 167)*

Following the completion of a training program, the assistant may engage only in those duties that are planned, designed, and supervised by the professional . . .

1. Screen speech, language, and/or hearing;

2. Implement evaluative or management programs and procedures that are
   a. planned and designed by the professional,
   b. included in published materials which have directions for administration and scoring and for which the aide has received training,
   c. specific clinical procedures for which the aide has been trained;

3. Record, chart, graph or otherwise display data relative to client performance;

4. Maintain clinical records;

5. Report changes in client performance to the professional having responsibility for that client;

6. Prepare clinical materials, including ear molds;

7. Test hearing aids to determine if they meet published specifications;

8. Participate with the professional in research projects, in-service training, public relations programs, or similar activities.

The assistant may not engage in any of the following activities:

1. Interpret obtained observations or data into diagnostic statements or clinical management strategies or procedures:

2. Determine case selection;

3. Transmit clinical information (including data or impressions relative to client performance, behavior, or progress) either verbally or in writing to anyone other than the professional;

4. Independently compose clinical reports except for progress notes to be held in the client's file;

5. Refer a client to other professionals or other agencies;

6. Use any title either verbally or in writing other than that determined by the professional. (pp. 167–168)*

---

*From the American Speech-Language-Hearing Association, Committee on Supportive Personnel, Guidelines for the Employment and Utilization of Supportive Personnel in Audiology and Speech-Language Pathology, *ASHA, 23*, 1981.

It may be helpful for student clinicians to know there has been some resistance in the speech-language field to the use of supportive personnel. The most common attitude has been that communication aides would limit the role of speech-language pathologists to that of diagnosticians; however, the literature supports the effectiveness of the communication aide. "Supportive personnel successfully expanded and supplemented the services of the speech and language specialist, providing a valuable contribution to the [school] speech and language program" (Scalero, 1976, p. 150). It is imperative, therefore, that student clinicians learn the importance of proper supervision of a communication aide so the aide may augment the speech-language services in ways beneficial to all concerned.

Learning to work successfully with a paraprofessional is a skill that many speech-language pathologists have found perplexing or difficult. Student clinicians will benefit by having an opportunity to work in a setting in which there is an aide or having an opportunity in a proseminar to discuss or role play the experience of working with a paraprofessional. Two areas of consideration are important when working with paraprofessionals: interpersonal relationships and giving directions.

To develop a peer relationship can invite a familiarity that may make it impossible for the speech-language pathologist to remain in charge. To become too friendly may make it difficult for the speech-language pathologist to direct the communication aide in fulfilling the needs of the pupils in the case load. To remain aloof may interfere with a cooperative relationship developing between the professional and the aide. Professional behaviors toward the communication aide enhance interpersonal relationships: (1) treat the communication aide as you would wish to be treated if you were in that position, (2) remember most communication aides are working for a salary and may be dependent on supporting themselves, (3) be considerate, (4) be supportive and give praise when deserved, (5) give assistance when warranted, (6) be friendly without crowding the aide's privacy or territory, (7) be sincere and willing to share, (8) be helpful without taking over the aide's work, and (9) expect from the aide a reasonable commitment to the job and a realistic interest in the field of speech-language pathology.

The performance of the communication aide is dependent upon the clinician's ability to give directions: (1) be specific and precise, (2) use language that is readily understood by a nonprofessional, (3) give few directions at one time, (4) be consistent, (5) develop written guidelines and refer to them frequently, (6) set due dates and give periodic reminders, (7) review procedures and, when appropriate, invite suggestions, and (8) give directions as positive statements avoiding contradictory phrases that may lead to misinterpretations.

During the school assignment, student clinicians may be involved for the first time in learning how to perform in a professional manner with paraprofessionals. This may be the first opportunity student clinicians have had to demonstrate to another adult their knowledge of speech-language pathology. The professional is expected to work efficiently with communication aides. This is a skill student clinicians should, if possible, develop during their student teaching experience.

Overview

As student teaching nears completion, it is helpful for student clinicians to step back and evaluate the assignment as a holistic experience. By viewing the *total* experience, they can review the activities in which they have participated and identify areas in which they need additional training. Student clinicians should be aware of the diversity of their experiences, but they should remember it is not possible for them to participate in every activity during this one assignment. Student clinicians usually become so involved in the day-to-day requirements of the assignment it is difficult for them to measure and evaluate the experiences they have had and the progress they have made. It is recommended that student clinicians *write* an overview of their student teaching experiences. The writing of an overview is a means of gaining objectivity, and it forces the student clinician to put events into proper perspective.

CONCLUSION

Success in student teaching has been discussed in its many aspects throughout this chapter. Figure 4 graphically shows those qualities which are essential for success: theoretical knowledge, clinical ability, interpersonal relationships, professional qualities, and self-assessment/self-evaluation.

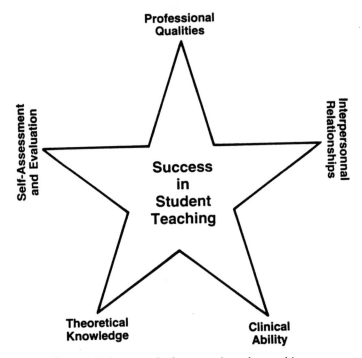

Figure 4. Major categories for success in student teaching.

After many months of preparation, students reach that point in their training when they must leave the sheltered environment of the academic setting for a whole new world. Student teaching is the transition from student status to professional standing. Peers no longer will be other students but will be experienced professionals from many backgrounds.

Although student teaching may be cause for anxiety and uncertainty, there is also a feeling of emergence. When a student has a sound academic and clinical background, a feeling of self-worth, and a positive feeling of expectancy toward the assignment, student teaching can be a stimulating and rewarding experience. ENJOY IT!

Chapter 4

THERAPEUTIC APPROACHES FOR THE ADOLESCENT WITH A COMMUNICATION PROBLEM

DOROTHY MCJENKIN

Although much attention has been given to the importance of providing services for the speech, hearing, and language impaired child, little has been written in the literature concerning the adolescent with a communication disorder. The student clinician may have limited experience in working with this age group and may view the assignment with uncertainty.

SELF-CONCEPT

The high school years are known for their influence on shaping the personality of the human being. At this time adolescents begin to separate from their parents and develop their own self-identity. They are self-conscious and full of uncertainty. It is during these years that teenagers acquire new values and begin the long process of finding themselves (Offer, 1969). The turbulent period of adolescence holds special problems for the pupil with a speech, hearing, and language disorder. These pupils are penalized in the highly verbal give and take of our classrooms today. They are isolated from their classmates and their friends as well. Their inadequacy in expressing themselves affects their schoolwork, their grades, and their relationships with others (Marge, 1965). A speech-language problem tends to undermine an individual's self-evaluation and personality adjustment (Palmer, 1964). These are individuals who have had problems in the area that hurts, the area of interpersonal relationships. Wherever there is a speech, hearing, or language problem, there is some degree of breakdown in communication. This breakdown leads to difficulties in interpersonal relationships, and the difficulties in interpersonal relationships lead to further breakdowns in communication. The speech-language pathologist can help break this vicious cycle by providing pupils with an opportunity to communicate with a person who accepts them totally as they are, but who views them as individuals who have the potential to make changes in their lives and in their communication skills.

RELATIONSHIPS WITH ADULTS AND PEERS

While adolescents may refuse to accept the ideas and directions of some adults, they are still able to identify with certain adults who do not represent the authority against whom they are rebelling (Black, 1960). The opinions of their peers can carry great weight and may even hinder them from facing their speech-language problems objectively. If speech-language therapy is perceived as an attempt to change them, teenagers will resist. If speech-language therapy is viewed as an opportunity to experiment with change under the guidance of an accepting, caring adult, then growth and change can take place. The speech-language pathologist must be prepared to interact *with* the pupils rather than *upon* them.

THE THERAPEUTIC RELATIONSHIP

Albert Murphy (1974) has stated that our persons are more important than our techniques. Speech-language pathologists working with high school pupils must first know, understand, and accept themselves. They must be in touch with their own feelings and open to the feelings of others. They must be aware of their own strengths and weaknesses and accepting of these in the teenagers as well. Adolescents need positive, affirming voices, and the speech-language pathologist must be able to provide a warm, therapeutic relationship in which there is empathy, an atmosphere of trust, acceptance, and mutual understanding. Speech-language therapy is an art as well as a skill, and speech-language pathologists must be prepared to be in touch with themselves, to listen to their own inner voices and rely on their clinical judgment.

High school pupils are quick to recognize a phony. Student

clinicians initially may feel uncomfortable in working with pupils so near their own age level. They may be reticent in approaching an individual in one to one therapy without some kind of gimmick or game. It helps to keep in mind that communication disordered adolescents do not need a twenty-two- or twenty-three-year-old friend, but rather a friendly therapist who can be objective in assisting them in attaining more effective communication skills. Trying to talk or dress as one of the gang is a sure way to turn teenagers off. Teenagers respond to knowing that therapists are also imperfect beings who are making themselves, their skills, and their experiences available to them. Speech-language pathologists who are at ease with themselves and in touch with their own feelings can create a climate in which the pupil is free to change. The adolescent years are fraught with changes. Since change can be a frightening thing, pupils need to realize that only they have the power to change themselves. Adolescents grow toward maturity as they assume the responsibility for their own actions and their own communication.

IMPLICATIONS FOR THERAPY

Motivation

Teenagers are keenly interested in themselves and painfully aware of others. It has been stated that all teenagers have the right to the three Bs: they need to *be* themselves, to *be*long to a group, to *be* recognized. Experiences that come from them can be the key to learning. Areas of interest from wrestling to roller skating can provide opportunities for discussion and communication. In order to motivate the pupils, the speech-language pathologist must find the teenagers' own areas of interest and strength and use them as the foundation for therapy. Stimulating materials that are of interest to young adults must be selected and used in such a way that they will build self-esteem and enhance teenagers in the eyes of their peers (Black, 1960). A positive comment about appearance or assets by the speech-language pathologist can help increase self-confidence in the pupil and "expand the area of the possible" (Maltz, 1960, p. 12). Adolescents are deeply interested in learning more about themselves, and this concern can be used as a basis for therapy.

Sense of Humor

Adolescents cannot stand oppressiveness. Therapy sessions are basically working sessions, but the tone needs to be light and not too serious. A good sense of humor is one of the most valuable tools the speech-language pathologist has in working with the teenager.

Objectivity and Flexibility

Teenagers live in a world of shifting moods. They are intensely preoccupied with themselves and acutely aware of others. They are full of self-doubt but may hide this through shifts of exhibitionism and withdrawal (Black, 1960). The speech-language pathologist must be prepared to deal with a world of black and white, to help the pupils define the problem and search for the alternative shades of gray. The speech-language pathologist should resist the temptation to give advice. Adolescents are told what to do by too many people. The speech-language pathologist must retain objectivity in assisting the pupils in finding their own solutions. Rather than trying to help with deep-seated problems that are beyond the speech-language pathologist's realm of training and expertise, referrals should be made to the properly trained professional. The speech-language pathologist also needs to be aware that what may appear to be a cataclysmic problem or disaster one week may have disappeared entirely from the horizon by the next session.

The speech-language pathologist must always be well prepared with a variety of appropriate materials designed to accomplish short-term goals, but a selection of alternative procedures should be available if planned activities do not appear to be working. Flexibility also means being able to drop a perfectly prepared lesson and deal with a pressing problem that needs immediate attention. Objectivity and flexibility are essential parts of the speech-language pathologist's approach.

THE HIGH SCHOOL AS A SETTING FOR
SPEECH-LANGUAGE THERAPY

High schools traditionally have been known to be subject oriented in contrast to elementary schools, which are pupil centered. Secondary schools are generally large and departmentalized and may be concerned with a variety of problems, such as truancy and drugs, which may seem more important than speech-language services. Nevertheless, it is up to the speech-language pathologist to be an effective communicator of the goals and purposes of speech-language services and how they fit into the total school program. It is not enough to be an effective speech-language pathologist within the confines of the speech-language therapy room. It is necessary to get out and be adept at spreading the word to the total school personnel.

How to Begin

Since the first few days of school can resemble a disaster center, the speech-language pathologist may appear totally unnecessary. Nevertheless, it is necessary to start. A place to begin is with introductions — to everyone.

Who's Who

Secretaries are key figures in the school world, and *principals' secretaries* need to view speech-language pathologists as people they know and are happy to see, not one more problem in a hectic day. Speech-language pathologists need to listen to them and let them know their school problems are a matter of interest and concern; they can be invaluable in assisting speech-language pathologists with their school needs, e.g. locating records, supplies, or an extra chair.

Principals are responsible for everything that goes on in their school. They will need to know the speech-language pathologist and the way the speech-language therapy program fits into the goals and philosophy of their school. They need to know *when* the speech-language pathologist is there, *why* the speech-language pathologist is there, *what* the speech-language pathologist is doing and with whom. Administrators are interested in having their faculty work in the best interest of the education for all the pupils. They need to know that the speech-language pathologist is an interested and willing member of their team.

The staff are important in implementing a successful program. As someone new to the school, it is up to the speech-language pathologist to make the first move. Secondary teachers have been well trained in particular areas of subject matter but may know little about speech-language therapy. Due to large class sizes and numerous classes, their opportunities to know individual students may be limited. Add to this that the speech, language and hearing disordered students are the silent ones, and the teachers may be totally unaware of the real communication problems of their pupils. As teachers, however, they are concerned about the pupil who does not participate in class, who may have a poor attitude and poor attendance, so they should be responsive to pooling resources with the speech-language pathologist to find out how better to meet the needs of these pupils.

It is up to speech-language pathologists to sell the program and themselves. It is important to talk at faculty meetings, to go to the teachers' lounge, to know the teachers, and see them in their rooms. Speech-language pathologists should remember that there are generally two lunch periods, so it is wise to alternate lunch hours when possible so that a broader range of contacts can be made in the teachers' lunch room. Speech-language pathologists should introduce themselves and remember teachers' names. Mrs. Jones may not remember the speech-language pathologist's name, but when Johnny begins stuttering in history class, she will know there is someone available to help him. One measure of how effective the person is in selling the program is how long the speech-language pathologist is viewed by the regular faculty as a substitute teacher!

Some special school personnel can be of assistance. In many schools the teachers who are respected the most by pupils are the coaches and leaders at sports activities (Offer, 1969). They have opportunities to know students individually and their opinions carry impact. They can be valuable allies, e.g. a coach may assign special duties to a communication disabled teenager; even sorting towels or keeping statistics can seem prestigious when accompanied by the special interest of the coach.

School nurses see pupils when they are the most vulnerable — when they are ill and in need of assistance. Communication problems are more likely to be apparent at this time. Health personnel can be important sources for referrals.

School psychologists offer assistance in advanced testing and help for pupils with emotional difficulties.

Girls and boys vice-principals are in contact with pupils who may need speech and language therapy. The speech-language pathologist may need their ears to put in a word for pupils in difficulty.

Counselors are concerned with individual pupils and their problems in meeting success in high school. They are trained professionals available for pupils in need and are a critical source of referrals.

Secretaries and custodians are the backbone of the school and can provide assistance in making the program run more smoothly.

Instructors in special education and learning disabled classes frequently have large numbers of pupils who are experiencing communication difficulties. These teachers generally welcome the assistance of the speech-language pathologist in improving pupils' communication skills. This ever-present case load can be drawn upon while some of the less obvious disabilities are being identified.

Communication aides in special education classrooms are also excellent resource contacts, since they are working closely with pupils on a day-to-day basis and are aware of the individual communication problems of these pupils.

In the initial stages it is helpful to make contact with one key person, perhaps a counselor, vice-principal or secretary, who can show the speech-language pathologist the ins and outs of how the school is run. Such items as hall passes for all pupils may seem routine to high school personnel, but these are generally unknown in an elementary setting, and the speech-language pathologist may be unfamiliar with their use. Young clinicians may have the unsettling experience of being asked for their hall passes as they are mistaken for pupils. Unfortunately this day passes all too soon!

DEVELOPMENT OF THE PROGRAM

Case Finding

The speech-language pathologist may find that one of the greatest challenges on the secondary level is locating the pupils. Most authorities agree that the most effective procedure for identifying pupils is the *survey* (Van Hattum, 1969). The initial conference with the principal should be used to explore which classes would be best to survey. Many speech-language pathologists test incoming freshmen in their English classes, since these classes are of a practical size, and English teachers are more closely allied to the field of speech communication. The speech-language pathologist contacts the administrator and describes the procedure used for speech and language surveying. The department chairperson is then contacted and a schedule of classes is obtained. A survey schedule is worked out and sent to the principal, department chairperson, and the teachers involved. Before the speech and language survey begins, a brief note should be sent to the instructor on the specifics of the survey, indicating that a quiet activity should be scheduled. The speech and language screening test may be administered in the back of the classroom or just outside the door. Surveying is a demanding task, so it is wise not to schedule screening tests for the entire day. It is possible to screen thirty to thirty-five pupils per period.

When the speech-language pathologist initiates the survey, it is wise to take a few minutes to talk to the entire class, introducing oneself and indicating this is not a test. A good first impression can be critical in letting pupils know that a warm, caring professional is enthusiastic about assisting them in polishing their communication skills. When conducting the survey, the speech-language pathologist can ask the pupils' names, have them count to ten, and talk to them briefly about themselves. The speech-language pathologist may want to have the pupils read some sentences designed to test specific speech sounds and assess some type of language processing. Having the pupils describe their best friend or an action picture can give the speech-language pathologist a more extensive speech and language sample when necessary. Results can be recorded on three-by-five cards with the pupil's name, disorder, severity, and decision whether therapy is necessary. It is important to report the results of the survey to the principal and teachers, indicating problems identified, decision whether therapy is necessary, and so forth. Although it is time-consuming, the survey lays the groundwork for expanding speech and language services so that they meet the needs of communication-disordered pupils in the entire school.

Referrals

Communication patterns can differ from situation to situation, so it is possible for pupils to pass the screening test and still be in need of speech and language therapy, e.g. a stutterer may be missed if there is limited time for conversation and the content is not emotionally ladened. The use of referrals by staff personnel is another method of identifying communication disabled pupils. Teachers, nurses, and counselors should be supplied with a simple form to fill out with the name of any pupil they feel could benefit from therapy. Particularly good sources of referrals are teachers of the developmentally disabled and the learning disabled, who may have a large number of pupils who need special help.

It is best not to send out referral forms earlier than two weeks after the start of school, preferably a month or so after. This gives the teachers an opportunity to know the pupils. If possible, the speech-language pathologist should introduce the referral form at a faculty meeting so instructors can associate a face with the referral. Referrals should be sent out periodically throughout the year so that the forms are less likely to get lost along the way. A referral should always be responded to promptly, and the results returned with a thank you to whoever referred the pupil. Some procedure should be worked out with counselors so that all pupils new to the school are screened by the speech-language pathologist. Pupils at this age also refer themselves. A notice can be placed in the daily bulletin stating the days the speech-language pathologist is there. The notice also may encourage pupils to ask their counselor for a pass to see the speech-language pathologist. Other sources of referral are the elementary or junior high school speech-language pathologists who are concerned about their former pupils receiving continued therapy. Cumulative records and health records also can be consulted to identify pupils with previously reported communication disorders.

Case Selection

After the survey has been completed and all referrals have been checked, the speech-language pathologist is ready to evaluate those pupils who are experiencing communication difficulties. Speech-language pathologists are mandated to provide services to communication handicapped children under PL 94-142, Education for All Handicapped Children Act. While determining their eligibility for the program based on test results, the speech-language pathologist also may want to be aware of the nature and severity of the speech and language problem on the teenagers' personality, education, and goals, and most important, their own evaluation of the need for speech and language therapy. Pupils who refer themselves are highly motivated, and this needs to be taken into consideration. Guidelines developed by the Los Angeles Unified School District (Hayes, 1969) to assist the speech and language pathologist in evaluating pupils include the following:

1. Degree of personal discomfort the problem is causing the student
2. Influence of impinging environmental and psychological factors on the student, i.e. parents, siblings, teachers, peers, self-image
3. How well the student can be understood by others
4. Student's awareness of his problem
5. Motivational level of the student, e.g. correction of speech problem, avoiding a scheduled class, pleasing parents, gaining attention
6. Evaluation of speech in terms of time spent in previous therapy
7. Overt physical abnormalities
8. Therapy from other agencies
9. Multiple factors, e.g. substandard speech, regional speech, bilingualism

10. Previously recorded data, e.g. cumulative record, health card, case history, test scores
11. Student's potential in relation to his stated vocational goals
12. Unusual and significant behavioral patterns
13. Growth and development in relation to age and sex

Scheduling

One of the biggest headaches in a high school program is scheduling. Just as the speech-language pathologist has everything nearly arranged, pupils change their schedule, and it is necessary to start all over. The speech-language pathologist must schedule around performance classes, lunches, assemblies, and most "solids." English teachers are generally receptive to pupils' using a portion of their class time for speech and language therapy, since this can be viewed as part of oral English. Pupils should know which classes they can best afford to miss, but they may need some guidance in this from the speech-language pathologist. Teachers are informed of the pupil's enrollment in speech and language therapy, and their cooperation is enlisted. It helps to have strong backing from the administration, who view speech and language services as important and vital to the educational success of the pupil. When this philosophy is expressed by the principal at preschool meetings, teachers frequently are more willing to tolerate the inconvenience of having pupils miss their classes. It also helps to indicate a willingness to adjust the schedule if there is a serious conflict. The instructors are notified that the pupil is expected to make up all class work missed and is not to be excused from tests. Sessions usually vary from thirty minutes twice a week to sixty minutes once a week.

Most work on the high school level is done with individual students. Adolescents and their communication problems are complex, and usually it is necessary to build strong one-to-one relationships with the speech-language pathologist before they are ready to identify with fellow students who also have communication problems. Groups can be employed when pupils are ready to practice newly learned communication skills with peers.

Grouping

Combining adolescents in groups for speech and language therapy takes a great deal of sensitivity and skill. Mental and emotional ages must be considered as well as physical appearance, personality factors, and the type of communication disorder. It helps to arrange to include at least one pupil who is attractive, friendly, and personable and who relates well to the speech-language pathologist and is someone with whom the pupils can identify (Black, 1960). A prominent athlete is almost sure to make the group successful!

Groups provide a vehicle for pupils to share feelings and ideas and encourage interaction and communication among teenagers. As the speech-language pathologist fosters mutual respect and regard for members of the group, as individual feelings and ideas are expressed and accepted, a feeling of warmth and solidarity grows and develops. Communication-disabled pupils are frequently weak in the area of interpersonal relationships, and groups provide an excellent opportunity to build friendships and promote improved communication patterns, which carry over outside the therapy setting.

Finding Space

The next problem is scheduling a room. Somehow there always seems to be a space shortage, but usually speech-language pathologists can find a conference room, a counselor's office, or a cubbyhole off the nurse's room. The best room is a small one with privacy for pupils coming and going. Unless sound treated, it should be located away from gymnasiums and music rooms.

Procedures for Getting the Pupils to Therapy

One of the best methods for calling pupils is to use a monitor or student help that is usually available in the attendance, guidance, or nurse's office. Reminders can be placed in the teacher's box on the day of therapy, but teachers are busy, and they may forget. Appointment cards or passes may be given to the pupils ahead of time, but they, too, forget, and the faithful do not need reminding.

The intercom is one of the least satisfactory methods of contacting pupils, since it broadcasts to the entire room what is a personal matter to the pupil. If absolutely necessary, call at the beginning or end of the period to avoid interruptions and attention. No one method works all the time, but a combination usually will.

What To Do If Pupils Do Not Come

Absenteeism can be a problem with communication-disordered pupils. They may be facing failure in their other classes, and it may take time before the relationship between the speech-language pathologist and pupils grow to the place where speech and language therapy is a vital and motivating force in teenagers' lives. Pupils who are consistently absent or late may be demonstrating patterns of resistance in accepting the responsibility of changing their speech and language behaviors. An objective review of their absence and tardy patterns may be needed, as well as a frank discussion of their commitment to the speech and language therapy program. The door should always be left open if they are not ready to pursue improving communication abilities at the present time.

Speech-language pathologists can use any vacant spots in their schedule to consult records, confer with teachers, nurses, and counselors, do additional evaluations, assist in audiometric screening, develop public relations, and so forth. If there has been a previous speech and language therapy program at the school, former pupils from last year's case load can be located and interviewed. Records kept or sent on ninth graders can be reviewed for pupils in need of service. Time can also be spent on keeping current records up-to-date.

Record Keeping

A systemic method of reporting and keeping records is an essential part of the secondary speech and language therapy program. Accountability means credibility. Some types of records needed include survey results, identification cards containing such information as name, age, sex, address, and telephone number, home room number, current class schedule, teachers' names, and indication of type and severity of speech, hearing, and language problem; case history with detailed information on health and medical history and test results; daily logs, indicating objectives of therapy sessions and results; and individual educational plans for each student, including present level of performance, assessment tools, long-range goals and short-range objectives, procedures and materials to be used, and end of semester evaluation and recommendations. Periodic reports should be sent to the administration regarding the number and types of cases served, as well as their progress.

Diagnosis and Remediation

Diagnosis must be ongoing. In the initial sessions rapport is established, and the speech-language pathologist sets the stage for a mutual discovery of the obstacles that are blocking the path to effective communication. A give-and-take approach that is centered around pupils' individual needs allow them to develop their own patterns for therapy, provided there are reasonable controls. These limits include the use of descriptive rather than evaluative assessment. It is preferable to say, "It sounds as if the air is coming out from the sides of your tongue," rather than, "You're not trying." Another limitation is one of complete privacy and reassurance that no information shared in the therapy session will be discussed outside of therapy without the pupil's permission. A third limit is that school rules are to be upheld during the therapy sessions.

Testing and diagnosis extend over several sessions and may begin with the speech-language pathologist obtaining factual information about the pupil: family history, previous schools, physical information, and so forth. These can put the pupils at ease because they are nonthreatening questions for which they have answers. The speech-language pathologist may want to skip an oral peripheral examination at this time, since pupils may be acutely self-conscious and feel uncomfortable with someone peering into their mouths. The speech-language pathologist must be well organized with all testing and have materials readily available. The purpose of each test should be explained, and the speech-language pathologist must be an active listener and a keen observer, e.g. such behaviors as gait, posture, and the way the student holds a pencil can all give indications of neurological integrity.

Listening Skills

Messages are transmitted not only by words but by tone, gesture, expression, and posture. Often this body language speaks more loudly and clearly than words. A doleful expression, a rigid posture can reveal a pupil's feelings before words are spoken. Just as an active listener takes the speaker's words and restates them so that there is no misunderstanding of meaning, speech-language pathologists may want to feed back to the pupil what they see as well as hear, e.g. "It seems like something is bothering you today." A relationship is only as good as its communication, so speech-language pathologists need to try to listen with their inner ear and transmit empathy, sensitivity, and understanding. They must accept, reflect, and clarify feelings, as well as ideas. Some helpful techniques include the use of open-ended statements, e.g. "Could you explain more fully what you mean?" clarifying and summarizing what has been expressed, e.g. "This is what I have been hearing," redirecting the student to the problem at hand when he has strayed far from the area of concern.

In sharing the results of diagnostic testing and setting up goals for therapy, speech-language pathologists must respect the pupil's autonomy. They may be concerned with what appears to be a mild lisp, while the speech-language pathologist has identified a pervasive problem in expressive language. It may be practicable to start with what they want to do and then lead them into other areas of concern. Evaluating together the pupil's total range of communication abilities, including strengths as well as weaknesses, can be profitable. These would include voice, fluency, language, and articulation skills (Ratkevich, 1975). Pointing out to pupils that they have pleasant voices and speak smoothly and easily may soften the difficulty of facing an unattractive lateral /s/ or an infantile /r/ problem. Speech-language pathologists are safe when they report observable behavior, and the pupil is able to accept that the pathologist is sharing the discovery of certain facets of the pupil's communication patterns.

TESTS

Articulation Tests

Austin Spanish Articulation Test, Learning Concepts. 2501 N. Lamar, Austin, TX 78705.

Fairbanks Sentence Articulation Test, *Voice and Articulation Drillbook,* Harper and Row, 10 East 53rd St., New York, NY 10022.

Fisher-Logeman Test of Articulation Competence, Houghton-Mifflin Co., 2 Park St., Boston, MA 02107.

Iowa Pressure Test, Counihan, D., Articulation skills of adolescents and adults with cleft palates, *J. Speech Hearing Disorders,* 25:181–187, 1960.

McDonald Deep Test of Articulation, Stanwix House, 3020 Chartiers Ave., Pittsburgh, PA 15204.

Photo Articulation Test, The King Company, 2414 Lawrence Ave., Chicago, IL 60625.

Auditory Discrimination and Perception Tests

Brown-Carlsen Listening Comprehension Test, Harcourt, Brace and World, Inc., 757 Third Ave., New York, NY 10017.

Goldman-Fristoe-Woodcock Auditory Skills Test Battery, American Guidance Service, Publishers' Building, Circle Pines, MN 55014.

Lindamood Auditory Conceptualization Test, Teaching Resources Corp., 100 Boylston, Boston, MA 02116.

Oliphant Auditory Synthesizing Test, Oliphant, G., Educators Publishing Service, Inc., 75 Moulton St., Cambridge, MA 02138.

Roswell-Chall Auditory Blending Test, Essay Press, P.O. Box 5, Planetarium Station, New York, NY 10024.

Screening Test for Auditory Perception, Academic Therapy Publications, Inc., 20 Commercial Blvd., Novato, CA 94947.

Wepman Auditory Discrimination Test, Language Associates, 175 E. Delaware, Chicago, IL 60611.

Language Tests

Apraxia Battery for Adults, Dabul, B., C.C. Publications, P.O. Box 23899, Tigard, OR 97223.

Assessment of Children's Language Comprehension (ACLC), Consulting Psychological Press, 577 College Ave., Palo Alto, CA 94306.

Bankston Language Screening Test, University Park Press, 233 East Redwood St., Baltimore, MD 21202.

Boston Diagnostic Aphasia Examination, Lea and Febiger (Pub.), 600 Washington Square, Philadelphia, PA 19106.

Clinical Evaluation of Language Functions, Charles Merrill, Publ. Co., 1300 Alum Creek Dr., Box 508, Columbus, OH 43216.

Language Sample—Written and Oral

Mecham's Verbal Language Development Scale, Western Psychological Associates, 12031 Wilshire Blvd., Los Angeles, CA 90025.

Minnesota Test for Differential Diagnosis of Aphasia, University of Minnesota Press, 2037 University Ave., S.E., Minneapolis, MN 55455.

Myklebust Picture Language Test, Western Psychological Associates, 12031 Wilshire Blvd., Los Angeles, CA 90025.

Porch Index of Communicative Ability, Consulting Psychologists Press, 577 College Ave., Palo Alto, CA 94306.

Revised Token Test, McNeil, M., University Park Press, 233 East Redwood St., Baltimore, MD 21202.

Specific Language Disabilities Test, Malcomesius, N., Educators Publishing Service, 75 Moulton St., Cambridge, MA 02138.

Test of Syntactic Ability, Quigley, S., Steinkamp, M., Power, D. and Jones, B., Dormac, Inc., P.O. Box 752, Beaverton, OR 97005.

Utah Test of Language Development, Communication Research Associates, P.O. Box 11012, Salt Lake City, UT 84147.

Verbal Power Test of Concept Equivalents, Western Psychological Associates, P.O. Box 775, Beverly Hills, CA 90213.

Wiig-Semel Test of Linguistic Concepts, Charles Merrill Publ. Co., 1300 Alum Creek Dr., Columbus, OH 43216.

Woodcock Language Proficiency Battery, English Form, Teaching Resources Corp., 100 Boylston, Boston, MA 02116 (for speakers of English as a second language).

Vocabulary Tests

Ammons Quick Test and *Ammons Full-Range Picture Vocabulary Test,* Psychological Test Specialists, Box 1441, Missoula, MT 59801.

Revised Peabody Picture Vocabulary Test, American Guidance Services, Inc., Publishers' Building, Circle Pines, MN 55014.

Stuttering Tests

Obtain baseline data on number and types of dysfluencies and secondary characteristics in reading phrases of increasing length, answering questions, and conversation.

Perceptions of Stuttering Inventory, Woolf, J., Assessment of stuttering as struggle, avoidance and expectancy, *British J. Disorders of Communication, 12*:158–171, 1967.

Personalized Fluency Control Therapy, Cooper, E., Learning Concepts, 2501 N. Lamar, Austin, TX 78705.

Scale of Communication Attitudes, Erickson, R., Assessing communication attitudes among stutterers, *J. Speech Hearing Research, 12*:711–724, 1969.

Stuttering Severity Instrument for Children and Adults, Riley, G., C.C. Publications, Inc., P.O. Box 23699, Tigard, OR 97223.

General Ability Tests

Gates Wide Range Achievement Test, Columbia University, 525 West 120th St., New York, NY 10027.

Peabody Individual Achievement Test, American Guidance Service, Publishers' Building, Circle Pines, MN 55014.

Hearing Tests

Barley CID Sentence Test, Jeffers, J. and Barley, M., *Speechreading (Lipreading),* Charles C Thomas, Publ., 2600 South First Street, Springfield, IL 62717. Hearing screening, air and bone conduction

Jean Utley Sentence Lipreading Test, Utley, J., *J. Speech Hearing Disorders, 11:*109–116, 1946.

Miscellaneous

Riley Motor Problems Inventory, Western Psychological Services, 12031 Wilshire Blvd., Los Angeles, CA 90025.

BOOKS AND MATERIALS

Speech and language therapy sessions, to be effective, must be centered around the interests and needs of the pupil. Areas of wide appeal should be considered, such as sports, humor, and current scientific events. One of the major decisions facing teenagers is a choice of vocation. In a short time they must decide whether to go on with their education or to seek employment. Many of them need assistance in exploring vocational opportunities and can profit from examining their own strengths and interests as they apply to future job possibilities. This is a good place to evaluate oral skills and decide what needs to be improved (Black, 1960). Units on career education are appropriate and meaningful in meeting the adolescent's need for self-knowledge and self-direction. Almost every teenager is vitally concerned with learning how to drive a car (virtually no one flunks driver's training!). The driver training manual can be a rich source of discussion and oral practice. Since there is a wide diversity of intellectual ability among pupils, it is critical to be aware of appropriate reading, language, and vocabulary levels. Teenagers are quickly turned off by material that is too low or too high for them.

The following books and materials may prove useful in working on the secondary level:

Action Books, Scholastic Magazine's Educational Challenges, Inc., 50 W. 44th St., New York, NY 10036. (Books geared to the secondary level with simple but interesting stories.)

Agnello, V. and Garcia, C., *A Workbook for Voice Improvement,* Interstate Printers and Publishers, 19-27 N. Jackson St., Danville, IL 61832.

Auditory Discrimination in Depth, Teaching Resources Corp., 100 Boylston Ave., Boston, MA 02116.

Barrios, A., *Towards Greater Freedom and Happiness,* Self-Programmed Control Center, P.O. Box 49939, Los Angeles, CA 90049. (Relaxation and biofeedback techniques useful in working with stutterers.)

Benagh, J., *Incredible Baseball Feats,* Grossett and Dunlop, 51 Madison Ave., New York, NY 10010. Paperback

Benagh, J., *Incredible Basketball Feats,* Grossett and Dunlop, 51 Madison Ave., New York, NY 10010. Paperback

Benagh, J., *Incredible Football Feats,* Grossett and Dunlop, 51 Madison Ave., New York, NY 10010. Paperback

Benagh, J., *Incredible Olympic Feats,* McGraw-Hill Book Co., Princeton Rd., Hightstown, NJ 08520.

Blockosky, V., Frazer, D. and Frazer, J., *30,000 Selected Words Organized by Letter, Sound and Syllables,* Communication Skill Builders, 3130 N. Dodge Blvd., Tucson, AZ 85733.

Boone, D., *The Voice and Voice Therapy,* Prentice-Hall, Englewood Cliffs, NJ 07632.

Brubaker, S. *Workbook for Aphasia,* Wayne State University Press, 5959 Woodward Ave., Detroit, MI 48202 (exercises for redevelopment of higher language functioning).

Bryngelson, B., *Know Yourself,* Burgess Publ. Co., 7108 Ohms Lane, Minneapolis, MN 55435 (a workbook for stutterers).

Building Safe Driving Skills, Texts and Workbooks, Fearon-Pitman Publ. Co., 6 Davis Dr., Belmont, CA 94002.

Bush, C., *Language Remediation and Expansion,* Reference List, Communication Skill Builders, 815 E. Broadway, P.O. Box 42050-G, Tucson, AZ 85733.

Bush, W. and Giles, M., *Psycholinguistic Aids to Teaching,* Charles Merrill Publ. Co., 1300 Alum Creek Dr., P.O. Box 508, Columbus, OH 43216.

Can of Squirms, A New Approach to Role Playing, Junior-Senior High School, Pennant Educational Materials, P.O. Box 20633, San Diego, CA 92120.

Cerf, B., *Houseful of Laughter,* Random House, Inc., 400 Hahn Rd., Westminster, MD 21157.

Chicago Board of Education, *A Speech Therapy Workbook,* Chicago, IL. (Material for discussion with stutterers along with exercises.)

Chrome Hand Counter, HC-1, Ideas, P.O. Box 741, Tempe, AZ 85281 (suited to count behavior rapidly).

Clarey, E. and Dixon, R., *Pronunciation Exercises in English,* Simon and Schuster, Inc., 1230 Ave. of the Americas, New York, NY 10020.

Copeland, M., *A Lipreading Practice Manual for Teenagers,* Alexander Graham Bell Assn. for the Deaf, 3417 Volta Place, N.W., Washington, DC 20007.

Development Language Materials; card sets: Photo Sequential Cards; Antonyms, Synonyms, Homonyms and Homophonic Cards; Reaction Cards; Written Language Cards; Story Telling Posters; Logic Cards; Functional Signs; Vocabulary Tracks; and Rhyming. Developmental Learning Materials, 7440 Natchez Ave., Niles, IL 60648.

Dixson, R., *Easy Reading Selections in English,* Simon and Schuster, Inc., 1230 Ave. of the Americas, New York, NY 10020.

Driver's Education for the Exceptional (film strips and tapes), Los Angeles City Unified School District, 450 N. Grand Ave., Los Angeles, CA 90071.

Drivers Education Manual, State Department of Motor Vehicles.

Dumont, L., *Consonant Articulation Drills,* Interstate Printers and Publishers, 19-27 No. Jackson St., Danville, IL 61832.

Fairbanks, G., *Voice and Articulation Drillbook,* Harper and Row Publ., Inc., E. 53rd St., New York, NY 10022.

Ferris, C., *Everyday Adventures and Updated Fables,* Charles Ferris, 8750 Paso Robles Ave., Northridge, CA 91324.

Feucht, R., *Vocabulary Development* (with word search puzzles, riddles and games), Hayes School Publishing Co. Inc., 321 Pennwood, Wilkinsburg, PA 13211.

Fisher, H., *Improving Voice and Diction,* Houghton-Mifflin Co., 2 Park St., Boston, MA 02107.

Flowers, A., *Big Book of Sounds,* Interstate Printers and Publishers, 19-27 N. Jackson St., Danville, IL 61832.

Flowers, A., *Language Building Cards,* Interstate Printers and Publishers, 19-27 N. Jackson St., Danville, IL 61832. (Originally designed for aphasic pupils, but adolescents in special education classes respond to them.)

Fokes Sentence Builder, Teaching Resources Corp., 100 Boylston, Boston, MA 02116.

Goda, S., *Articulation Therapy and Consonant Drillbook,* Grune and Stratton, 111 Fifth Ave., New York, NY 10003.

Gordon, M., *Speech Improvement,* Prentice-Hall, Englewood Cliffs, NJ 07632. (Auditory discrimination and articulation excercises with third to fourth grade reading level, but designed for young adult interest.)

Guiness Book of World Records, Bantam Books Inc., 666 Fifth Ave., New York, NY 10019.

Herr, S., *Program of Perceptual Communication Skills, Developing Auditory Awareness,* Instructional Materials and Equipment Distributors, 1520 Cotner Ave., Los Angeles, CA 90025.

Job Box, The, Fearon-Pitman Publ. Inc., 6 Davis Dr., Belmont, CA 94002.

Keith, R., *Speech and Language Rehabilitation: A Workbook for the Neurologically Impaired,* Interstate Printers and Publishers, 19-27 North Jackson St., Danville, IL 61832.

Kelly, J., *Clinicians Handbook for Auditory Training,* Volta Bureau, 3417 Volta Place, N.W., Washington, DC 20007.

Kilpatrick, K., *Therapy Guide for the Adult with Language and Speech Disorders,* Vol. 1 and 2, Visiting Nurse Service of Summit County, 1200 McArthur Dr., Akron, OH 44320. (Volume 2 has advanced level stimulus materials.)

Kramer, J., *Stuttering, Let's Talk it Over,* National Stuttering Project, P.O. Box 33, Walnut Creek, CA 94596. (Humorously written and illustrated booklet that can be used for discussion.)

Larr, A., *Tongue Thrust and Speech Correction*, Fearon-Pitman Publ. Co., 6 Davis Dr., Belmont, CA 94002.

Leavitt, J., *Stop, Look and Write*, Bantam Books, Inc., 666 Fifth Ave., New York, NY 10019.

Lipreading Practice Manual, Indiana Speech and Hearing Center, Indianapolis, IN.

Luter, J. and Modisett, N., *Speaking Clearly*, Burgess Publ. Co., 7108 Ohms Lane, Minneapolis, MN 55435.

MacNutt, E., *Hearing with Our Eye*, A Lipreading Textbook for Jr. High School Students, Volta Bureau, 3417 Volta Place, N.W., Washington, DC 20007.

Mayer, L., *Voice and Diction*, Wm. C. Brown Co. Publ., 2460 Kerper Blvd., Dubuque, IA 52001.

McKee, B., *Phonemic Approximation, R and S*, Bob McKee, 3415 Ione, Los Angeles, CA 90068.

Mowrer, D., *Program to Increase Fluency*, Ideas, P.O. Box 741, Tempe, AZ 85281.

Myklebust, H. and Johnson, D., *Learning Disabilities*, Grune and Stratton, 111 Fifth Ave., New York, NY 10003.

Nemoy, E. and Davis, S., *Correction of Defective Consonant Sounds*, Expression Co., P.O. Box 153, Londonderry, NH 03053.

Nilsen, D. and Nilsen, A., *Pronunciation Contrasts in English*, Regents Publ. Co., Inc., 2 Park Ave., New York, NY 10016.

Parnell, E., *Oxford Picture Dictionary of American English*, Oxford University Press, Inc., 200 Madison Ave., New York, NY 10016.

Polow, N., *Symptomatic Voice Therapy*, Modern Education Corp., P.O. Box 721, Tulsa, OK 74101.

Powell, J., *Why Am I Afraid to Tell You Who I Am?* (grade 7 through adult), Pennant Education Material, P.O. Box 20633, San Diego, CA 92120.

Price, R. and Stern, L., *Mad Libs*, Price, Stern, Sloan Publ., 410 N. La Cienega Blvd., Los Angeles, CA 90048.

Randall, F., *Getting A Job*, Fearon-Pitman Publ. Co., 6 Davis Dr., Belmont, CA 94002.

Schwartz, M., *Stuttering Solved*, J. B. Lippincott Co., 521 Fifth Ave.,

New York, NY 10017.

Scott, L. and Thompson, J., *Speech Ways*, Webster Publ. Co., 1221 Ave. of Americans, New York, NY 10020.

Shames, G., and Florance, C., *Stutter Free Speech*, Charles E. Merrill Publ. Co., 1300 Alum Creek Dr., P.O. Box 508, Columbus, OH 43216.

Smith, C., *Auditory Memory Training Exercises and More Auditory Memory Exercises.* (for children and adults), Volta Bureau, 3417 Volta Place, N.W., Washington, DC 20007.

Sobol, D., *Two Minute Mysteries*, Scholastic Book Services, 50 W. 44th St., New York, NY 10036.

Spill and Spell, No. 101, Philips Publishing Co., 1562 Main St., Springfield, MA 01103.

Stennett, N., *A Workbook for Stutterers*, Nadine Stennett, Grant Union School District, Sacramento, CA.

Streng, A., *Syntax, Speech and Hearing*, Grune and Stratton, 111 Fifth Ave., New York, NY 10003.

The $10,000.00 Pyramid Game, Milton Bradley (age 10 to adult).

Therapy for Stutterers, Speech Foundations of America, 152 Lombard Rd., Memphis, TN 38111. (This book is concerned with therapy for the older adolescent and adult stutterer.)

The Ungame, Pennant Educational Materials, P.O. Box 20633, San Diego, CA 92120. (Deals with communication problems, and helps players begin exploring their own feelings, attitudes, and motives.)

Understanding Our Feelings, Instructo No. 1215, Instructo Corp., Cedar Hollow & Mathews Rds., Paoli, PA 19301.

Using the Want Ads, Janus Book Publ., 2541 Investment Blvd., Hayward, CA 94545.

Whitehurst, M., *Integrated Lessons in Lipreading and Auditory Training.* Basic integrated material for hard of hearing adults and teenagers, Volta Bureau, 3417 Volta Place, N.W., Washington, DC 20007.

Word Making Cards, Word Making Productions, 70 W. Louise Ave., Salt Lake City, UT 84115.

Word Poppers; Sets I and II: Basic Sight Vocabulary, Sight Phrase Card, The Syllable Game, and Know Your States. Garrard Publ. Co., 107 Cherry St., New Canaan, CT 06840.

Working Makes Sense, Fearon-Pitman Publ. Co., 6 Davis Dr., Belmont, CA 94002.

World Traveler, Box 3618, Washington, DC 20007. (Ten issues per school year. A sixteen page full color magazine with an adult format useful in training and rehabilitation of teenagers and adults with speech and language disorders including aphasics and developmentally disabled.)

Zickefouse, W., *Oral Myo-Therapy Manual,* Oral Myo-Therapy Materials, 3165 Delwood Way, Sacramento, CA 95821.

TECHNIQUES

Techniques must take into consideration the cognitive abilities of teenagers and their need for a direct, open approach to therapy. If this is based on a nurturing client-therapist relationship, then the techniques can be effective.

A few favorite techniques include the following:

PROBLEM SOLVING APPROACH. Define the problem; explore the alternatives; decide on a course of action to take. Do not be afraid to make mistakes. Reevaluate, realizing there is no perfect solution, e.g. explain that diagnostics will help find what the problem is. Set up mutually agreed upon goals. Talk about how to get there and what approach sounds best. Can the pupils name the steps necessary to get there (placing the responsibility on them)? Reevaluate periodically to see if they are getting where they want to go. If it is not working, try something else.

SIMULATE THE SPEECH DIFFICULTY. Simulate as closely as possible their speech problem. Try to find out exactly what they are doing by duplicating tongue position, vocal quality, and so forth. Somehow, because someone is interested and cares enough to simulate their speech patterns, this adds to the building of a strong interpersonal relationship.

ROLE PLAYING. Simulated real-life situations can be used to prepare for job interviews, social situations, facing authority figures, and so forth. Write a script and tape-record it, playing it back to analyze articulation, language, fluency, and so forth.

TAPE RECORDER. Discussions can be recorded and replayed, with pupils responsible for noticing elements that are interfering with intelligibility, e.g. omitted endings, distorted sibilents, etc.

PHONIC MIRROR.® The excellent fidelity and automatic replay on the machine provides instant feedback and makes it an excellent tool for articulation and voice therapy.

LANGUAGE MASTER.® Visual and auditory feedback assists pupils in acquiring language concepts, and they enjoy the power of manipulating the machine themselves.

VIDEOTAPING. This technique provides eye opening feedback as to the total gestalt of the pupil's communication ability and the speech-language pathologist's as well!

PREDICTING ERRORS. In the carry-over stage, have pupils work against a timer to predict how many errors they will make in a certain period of time. Working against time pressure can also assist in strengthening responses and help in carry-over.

HOMEWORK ASSIGNMENTS. Rather than telling the pupils what and when to practice, have them decide how much they can practice, when they can practice, and with whom. They are the ones who know what is going on in their lives, and this gives them the responsibility for making the necessary changes in their communication patterns. Use the *contract* system for making assignments. Have them agree about their goals and sign for what they agree to carry out. Make provisions for documentation, such as charts, checklists, daily logs, or journals.

LANGUAGE. For oral language use story starters, material placed on index cards that may include discussion topics, such as weekends, or something I would like to change, things to describe, such as a person that you admire, a sport that you like, a problem to be solved, a situation to be explained. (Discussion topics shared by Mary Leonard.) For written language, try solving problems from "Dear Abby." The problems presented in this column are frequently of interest to teenagers and are those with which they can identify.

ARTICULATION. Phonemic approximation utilizing the /t/ preceding the /s/ can assist in gaining correct placement for a lateral /s/. Holding a mirror below the lower lip can give visual clues as to the width of the breath stream as it clouds the mirror. A straw also can be used to help direct the breath stream in a narrow, precise fashion. A toothpick can be used to stimulate the groove necessary for a sharper production of the sound. The adolescent usually can accept a direct type of drill approach and responds to experimentation.

MIRROR WORK. Teenagers may not be able to tolerate work with a full face mirror but usually can accept pocket mirrors where they can focus only on the mouth, teeth, and other articulators.

VOICE. When working with pupils who speak in a monotone, have them read magazine advertisements as if they were selling the product or make up a television commercial. This is tape-recorded and replayed for evaluation. Advertisements are conversationally written and are meant to be persuasive, which requires greater use of inflection for the pupil to sell the speech-language pathologist on the product.

STUTTERING. Use *The Ungame* for pupils who need to get in touch with their feelings. This uncompetitive and unthreatening game provides an opportunity for the speech-language pathologist to set an example in being open and honest and aids the pupil in feeling safe in sharing and becoming aware of feelings.

CONCLUSION

In working with teenagers, speech-language pathologists have the opportunity to accept them the way they are and to assist them in becoming what they want to be. One grows psychologically by encountering a difficulty and mastering it. One grows by solving problems. The speech-language pathologist can help adolescents realize that they have the freedom of choice—to remain static and do nothing about their lives or to take action and experiment with change, to grow through improving their communication skills.

It has been said that there are no rules about leaping into the unknown, since no one has ever been there before. For the speech-language pathologist just beginning work with the teenager, the most important ingredients to take along are a good listening ear, a sense of self-worth, patience, acceptance, flexibility, and humor. To work with adolescents is not easy, but the opportunity to challenge them through communication is an experience not to be missed.

PART II

THE ON-SITE SPEECH-LANGUAGE
PATHOLOGIST

OVERVIEW:

SIDE TWO OF THE TRIAD

Part II is written for the second member of the TRIAD, the speech-language pathologist employed in the school setting. Most speech-language pathologists take pride in their profession and many have a desire to be involved in shaping the profession. This may be attained through participation with students who are enrolled in university training programs. There are two ways in which speech-language pathologists in the schools participate in training students:

1. They make observations of therapy sessions available for students-in-training.
2. They accept a student clinician for the student teaching practicum.

Many speech-language pathologists are willing and eager to fulfill their professional responsibilities and seek a closer relationship with university programs, but they may not know what their role is in relation to the university training program. Part II of this text describes the role and responsibilities of on-site speech-language pathologists who cooperate with training institutions by offering observation opportunities for students-in-training or by accepting student clinicians for their school practicum experience.

Chapter 5 discusses the relevance of observations as an introduction for the student to the uniqueness, the potential, and the realities of speech-language programs in the schools. Students-in-

training considering this environment for professional employment gain valuable information to aid them in planning their
future goals. The emphasis of the chapter is on the role of the
speech-language pathologist in preparing for and managing observation assignments.

Chapter 6 discusses the purpose of being a master clinician and
details the role and responsibilities of speech-language pathologists
who accept this professional commission. Most speech-language
pathologists have only their own experience with their former
master clinicians to draw upon for information in fulfilling their
supervisory role. Although this may be an adequate base for
many speech-language pathologists, most master clinicians want
additional guidance to perform competently in this assignment.

Chapter 6 describes qualifications for being a master clinician.
Guidelines are included on how to be an effective master clinician
for students-in-training. Responsibilities, evaluation of students-
in-training, conferences with students and university personnel,
and participation in university activities are discussed in the
chapter. Modes, interactions, and relationships pertinent to the
supervisory role are discussed by Anderson (1974), Oratio (1977),
and Schubert (1978), and readers are referred to these sources
for supplementary information.

Chapter 7 is unique in that it describes speech-language-hearing
programs at the community college level. As a result of federal and
state legislation mandating services for the handicapped, more
and more community colleges are implementing speech-language-
hearing programs. Inasmuch as this is a new environment for
speech-language pathologists, little information has been published
in this area. This chapter discusses developing and implementing
a speech-language-hearing program in a community college.

Chapter 5

ON-SITE OBSERVATIONS

PURPOSE OF OBSERVATIONS

The strength of a viable profession is dependent upon experienced personnel in the field passing their knowledge and expertise to the next generation of new clinicians. Building on past achievements and preparing for future growth and expansion is the hallmark of ongoing professional commitment. This is the base for preserving the established standards of a profession while making it possible for continuing development to ensue. Speech-language pathologists by nature are caring individuals who find personal and professional satisfaction in sharing their skills and knowledge with others. Practicing speech-language pathologists have benefited from the experience of those who preceded them and take professional pride in being able to assist others who are now entering the field.

The total training of speech-language pathologists cannot be accomplished by university faculty alone. Speech-language pathologists in the field who give of themselves in this endeavor contribute an added dimension to students in training programs. University training programs can only introduce students to the profession. It is practicing speech-language pathologists who initiate them into the professional realities of the work environment.

Usually the first step a student takes into an actual work setting is through the mode of observations. On-site speech-language pathologists, remembering when they were students, can relate to the significance observations have for students-in-training. The on-site speech-language pathologist contributes to the professional growth of the students by making it possible for them (1) to see individuals with speech-language disorders receiving remediation, (2) to see group dynamics in action, (3) to see administrators, allied professionals, and paraprofessionals fulfilling their roles, and (4) to visit professional sites and see the facilities, furnishings, equipment, and materials available.

On-site speech-language pathologists understand one purpose of observations is to enable students-in-training to see children and adults with the types of speech and language disorders discussed in the university classroom setting. Often the on-site speech-language pathologist is the first to introduce students to a person exhibiting a communication disorder. In this experience students see that the simple articulation defect described in a textbook becomes a person. They are exposed to the Down's syndrome child, whose faulty language and articulation cause problems with intelligibility, or the cleft palate child whose nasal emission of sounds distorts vocal production. As discussed in Chapter 2, students are seeing unique *individuals* manifesting the symptoms previously studied and receiving therapy to remediate their communication disorder.

Frequently students have a theoretical background in group dynamics, but their actual experience in being with a group of children in a remediation situation may be limited. A classroom discussion of group dynamics is different from sitting in a room watching this process in action. Being in a position to observe directly children interacting with their peers and with the speech-language pathologist may be an exciting experience for students-in-training. This is textbook information becoming truly meaningful as it occurs in a real-life situation.

On-site speech-language pathologists can give students an inside view of other professionals carrying out their assigned roles in the best interests of those with a communication handicap. Students have heard and read how speech-language pathologists relate and interact with other on-site personnel to insure the clients the most comprehensive service possible. Students-in-training are currently in the position of being in an academic environment that by the nature of its objectives, is student oriented, whereas off-campus professional sites are client oriented. It is important, therefore, for students-in-training to be in a setting where the personnel share the common primary purpose of helping clients succeed in the challenging process of learning.

Students-in-training benefit from having the opportunity to

visit a number of different types of professional settings and to observe experienced speech-language pathologists function within each of these environments. Each site is a unique entity, and on-site speech-language pathologists have the opportunity to describe their particular facilities, furnishings, equipment, and materials. Students-in-training see how these vary from one site to another. What is important for students to learn is that highly professional services are performed within each of these distinct types of structures.

Most speech-language pathologists are receptive toward having observers from a university when it is convenient and practicable; however, there may be situations, children, and facilities that make observations impractical. Granting observation privileges to students in training programs is based ultimately on the policy of the school district, clinic, or hospital facility. When possible, most speech-language pathologists make themselves and their settings available to student observers.

Observations by students from university programs can be a stimulating experience for speech-language pathologists. For many, it is a means by which they keep current with what is taking place in university training programs. It is a way of actively participating in the training of future colleagues in the field of communication disorders. Observations provide contact with university faculty as well as the student population. For some speech-language pathologists, it is an avenue employed for publicizing their program and the experiences it offers as an off-campus practicum. For others, it is utilized to show their clinical skills, facilities, and clientele.

Inasmuch as professionals in the field of communication disorders frequently work in an isolated setting, that is, independently and often physically removed from their colleagues, they have a desire and need for feedback. Observations bring them into contact with individuals who have at least basic exposure to the field and share a common interest in the profession. Observations provide a modicum of feedback to on-site speech-language pathologists regarding their professional performance.

The on-site speech-language pathologist is offering a service and opportunity to the university training program and students-in-training. Although the on-site speech-language pathologist may be fulfilling a professional commitment, there are clinical advantages to be gained by having observers.

1. Speech-language pathologists and clients frequently are more motivated when there is a visitor in the session. A change from the usual routine' often provides additional stimulation for the session to move at a more productive rate.

2. Clients have a chance to show their newly acquired skills to the interested observer, thus providing the speech-language pathologist with an additional remediation technique.

3. Speech-language pathologists have an opportunity to demonstrate their techniques and materials. Generally the creative clinician is in great demand by student observers — word travels fast on university campuses. This response by students is favorable feedback to speech-language pathologists about their effectiveness as clinicians.

4. Speech-language pathologists may see themselves through the eyes of another, thus becoming more conscious of themselves as clinicians, of their pupils, and of the setting in which they work.

5. When there is only one speech-language pathologist on-site, there is an opportunity to interact with another individual in the field of communication disorders. When time allows, the speech-language pathologist may enjoy the opportunity to discuss cases and techniques with someone who has a background in the field.

6. Administrators and allied personnel become aware of the speech-language pathologist having the respect of colleagues when requests are received for observations.

PLANNING THE OBSERVATION

The conscientious speech-language pathologist is interested in providing the student observer with the most meaningful experience possible. The type of information speech-language pathologists receive in advance enables them to plan the observation period so that students gain the desired experiences. Speech-language pathologists should be aware that beginning students may not have sufficient background to know the potential of the experiences available at the setting; therefore, they may not be specific when requesting an observation.

The most meaningful experience takes place if the speech-language pathologist has some questions in mind when the observation is being planned with the student. Specific information will aid the speech-language pathologist to arrange the most beneficial observation:

1. Name of student and way to contact student in the event the observation must be cancelled
2. Purpose of the observation
3. Name of university training program, course for which observation is required, and name of the instructor
4. Type of clients to be observed
5. The way the student is to use the observation: class presentation, written report, research project, and so forth
6. Level of training and experiences the student has had regarding professional settings and special programs, i.e. has student previously observed secondary pupils at a special education site for the autistic
7. Date and length of observation

The speech-language pathologist may wish to give the student some special instructions in advance of the visit inasmuch as there may not be time on the day of the observation. Directions may include the following:

1. Designating the parking area
2. Specifying arrival time
3. Informing student where to meet, i.e. office, therapy room, lounge, or parking lot
4. Advising student to sign in at the office before coming to the therapy room
5. Asking the observer to refrain from note taking if it will be distracting to pupils
6. Requesting student observer to respond with appropriate behavior if an unforeseen situation arises, e.g. if a client becomes angry and upset, student observer may be expected or asked to leave the room

7. Requesting student observer to be prepared for introductions to the pupils and plan to interact with them as opportunities arise, or the converse, *not* to become involved with the clients

The speech-language pathologist is not solely responsible for making the observation a successful experience. It is a cooperative venture, which includes the joint efforts of the student and the university faculty. University faculty are responsible for defining clearly to students the purpose of the observation, explaining the behaviors they are to focus on, describing how they are to record pertinent information, and so forth. The role and participation of student observers are discussed in Chapter 2.

RESPONSIBILITIES

When speech-language pathologists agree to participate in the off-campus training of students, they are assuming certain responsibilities for those students. On-site speech-language pathologists become a model professional in the eyes of the student-in-training and are expected to demonstrate professional competence and etiquette.

Students-in-training expect to see professional performance, which combines a sound theoretical base with clinical expertise. They anticipate observing a professional who imparts confidence, motivation, and understanding to speech and language handicapped individuals. Students look forward to seeing an experienced speech-language pathologist who is knowledgeable, is capable, and exhibits pleasure in working in the profession.

Student requisites are usually minimal, but they are important, and most speech-language pathologists show professional etiquette when helping students-in-training fulfill their required assignments. Students are under pressure to submit assignments by due dates, and they are frustrated when they do not receive a return call from the on-site speech-language pathologist. When observations must be cancelled, the considerate on-site speech-language pathologist notifies students as soon as possible or attempts to find another site for them to use for observation. Otherwise, students are penalized for turning in late observation reports when, in fact, they were at the mercy of a person who neglected to inform them of the necessity for a change in plans. Being aware of these student needs is a demonstration of professional interest by the considerate speech-language pathologist.

CONCLUSION

When a speech-language pathologist agrees to accept student observers, a commitment is made to the profession, the site, the university program, and the student. Speech-language pathologists have the responsibility to present themselves as professionals worthy of being observed. They represent the profession by giving students additional insight into the field and by demonstrating the application of ethical practices. Speech-language pathologists represent the site by showing the student observer the facilities, describing the strengths of the speech-language program, discussing plans for new program directions, explaining the role of allied professionals, and presenting a realistic assessment of the program. By accepting student observers, speech-language pathologists are participating in the training of students; therefore, there is a responsibility to see that students have a meaningful observation to enrich the instruction provided on campus by the university.

Chapter 6

ON-SITE SUPERVISION OF
STUDENT CLINICIANS

M aster clinicians bring their experience as public school
speech-language pathologists to the second side of the student teaching TRIAD. When school speech-language pathologists
choose to assume the role of master clinician, they are committing
themselves to an additional professional responsibility. Their first
responsibility continues to be to the school district in which they
are employed, and their first priority must be to the children they
are hired to serve; therefore, it is necessary for them to effect a
balance in carrying out their obligations to both their pupils and
to their student clinicians.

First-time master clinicians frequently ask, "What is expected of
me?" The responsibilities of master clinicians and guidelines to
aid in this role are discussed in this chapter.

PURPOSE OF BEING A MASTER CLINICIAN

The basic purpose of being a master clinician is to provide a
student with an opportunity for on-the-job training. The master
clinician, as one side of the TRIAD, becomes an integral part of the
training program by expanding the student clinician's horizons from
campus clinic to the school environment. As a master clinician,
the school speech-language pathologist (1) teaches the educational
model, (2) introduces students to the practical application of clinical
speech and language in public education, (3) provides student clinicians with an opportunity to improve and strengthen clinical skills,
(4) functions as a supervisor, and (5) acts as an evaluator.

Student teaching is multipurposed. It provides students with an
opportunity (1) to learn how to function competently in the school
environment, (2) to improve and strengthen clinical skills, (3) to
meet state certification and professional association requirements,
(4) to be exposed to new situations and experiences, and (5) to

accumulate additional clinical hours.

It is imperative that student clinicians learn how the speech-language pathologist fits into the total educational model. Since the primary function of the schools is to educate large numbers of pupils, student clinicians must understand their objective is to aid children in achieving their educational potential. To help student clinicians function within the school setting, the master clinician does the following:

1. Discusses with the student clinician curriculum requirements for the various grade levels
2. Explains the chain of command within the school and district
3. Clarifies how accountability is to be documented
4. Describes record keeping procedures
5. Explains the administrative policies of the district and school
6. Teaches the student clinician how to implement state codes of education
7. Discusses federal laws affecting education for the handicapped, including mainstreaming
8. Discusses professional ethics

Student clinicians have spent the major portion of their academic lives learning theoretical concepts and acquiring clinical experiences in the university environment. It is the master clinician who introduces the student to the practical application of speech-language pathology in public education — how to organize a school speech and language program, how to function as part of an educational team, how to screen large numbers of children, and how to select a case load. Although the student has heard about many of the activities that are unique to a school setting, it is the master clinician who acts as a guide for the novice student clinician by introducing the student to the 8 AM to 3 PM work day — scheduling pupils for evaluation and therapy, conducting group and individual therapy sessions, participating in teacher and parent conferences, and so forth. As the student progresses in the assignment, the master clinician allows more of the daily responsibilities to be handled by the student, and eventually it is the student clinician who makes clinical judgments regarding the children in the case load.

Master clinicians are selected because of professional expertise; therefore, they are models for student clinicians. Master clinicians also are on-site supervisors, establishing direction, giving suggestions, and assisting and guiding students toward becoming independent professionals in a school setting. Several books and articles on the topic of supervision have been published. For information on supervision, the reader is referred to Anderson (1974), Oratio (1977), and Schubert (1978), and the extensive bibliographies cited by these authors.

A master clinician evaluates the performance of the student clinician, which requires a judgment to be made of the professional competence of an emerging speech-language pathologist. The evaluation serves a multipurpose function. It requires the master clinician to structure and formalize in writing the performance of the student clinician. A formal evaluation gives detailed feedback to the student regarding performance and level of competency. It also informs prospective employers of the level of competence that the student achieved in this experience and the potential ability of the student as a future professional speech-language pathologist.

Why does a school speech-language pathologist agree to assume the role of master clinician? Why should someone who has a full case load, Individualized Education Programs to write, parent conferences to initiate, in-service meetings to conduct, and school assessment team meetings to attend agree to take a student clinician, thereby willingly accepting an additional obligation? The reason so frequently emphasized in publications and conferences is that it is a responsibility that professionals are expected to assume. In reality, the reasons are varied and probably as individual as each master clinician. For some, it is the excitement of sharing the school experience with someone just starting in the field. It could be satisfaction with their own student teaching experience. For others, it could have been a poor student teaching assignment and the desire that another student should not encounter such negative experiences. Some school speech-language pathologists find themselves in an isolated environment, and the stimulation of sharing with another person in the profession may be the reason for accepting a student clinician. Many feel it is a compliment to be recognized by the university faculty or district supervisors as being an outstanding clinician. Some have special assignments that they find particularly exciting, and they may use this opportunity to publicize specialized areas, such as deaf, learning disabled, and autistic. The one reason seldom given is remuneration from the training institution. This is fortunate because few training programs, especially state universities, pay more than a token reimbursement to master clinicians.

It is acknowledged that accepting a student increases the work load of a school speech-language pathologist, but there are benefits to be derived by becoming a master clinician. Some of the benefits that the master clinician gains are (1) contact with the university training program, (2) exchange of current information (research, materials, etc.) from university to school setting and from school setting to the university program, (3) close association with university faculty, (4) input to the training program by way of ideas and suggestions that may influence training of future students, and (5) an opportunity to recruit competent school speech-language pathologists from the student teaching ranks.

Master clinicians have a lasting influence on the students they help train. Each of us who has been in a student teaching assignment undoubtedly remembers vividly our own master clinician, whose influence helped shape our attitude and approach to school therapy. Many of the student teaching remembrances are positive, but even the negative ones can be viewed as valuable learning experiences.

As with any new assignment, first-time master clinicians need to seek help in clarifying their role as part of the student teaching training team. Through talks with the university supervisor, in-service meetings, and discussions with experienced master clinicians, newly selected master clinicians begin to delineate their areas of responsibility. As new master clinicians begin to comprehend their roles, they understand better the roles of the other two members of the TRIAD: the student clinician and the university supervisor (see Chap. 3 and 9). "Practice makes perfect" and "the first experience is the hardest" are adages frequently applied to becoming a master clinician. It is through experience that master clinicians establish for themselves a frame of reference to apply to the performance of student clinicians.

Speech-language-hearing associations in some states have special interest groups whose purpose is to define the role of master clinicians and to urge greater recognitions of the contribution they make to the training of students. Master clinicians may find it beneficial to join such a group. If a state or regional group has not been established, innovative master clinicians may wish to form one within a geographical area or within the state association.

QUALIFICATIONS FOR MASTER CLINICIANS

Public school certification laws in each state establish minimum requirements for school speech-language pathologists. Employment in the schools legally qualifies speech-language pathologists to help train student clinicians from university programs; however, there are no established requirements for becoming a master clinician beyond state certification of speech-language pathologists in the schools. Some university programs and school districts have established minimum criteria that school speech-language pathologists must meet before they are assigned student clinicians. The absence of established state or national criteria, however, results in a lack of uniformity in qualifications for becoming a master clinician. Based on input from a large number of master clinicians, the following professional and personal qualifications are recommended:

Professional

1. Public school certification in language-speech-hearing
2. Master's degree in speech-language pathology or related area
3. State license in speech-language pathology in those states in which licensing has been legislated
4. American Speech-Language-Hearing Association Certificate of Clinical Competence in Speech-Language Pathology
5. Minimum of three years recent experience as a school speech-language pathologist
6. Clinical expertise
7. Clinical experience with pupils demonstrating a wide variety of language, speech, and hearing problems

8. Clinical experience with pupils of various ages from primary grades through junior high level, experience with preschoolers and high school students is desirable
9. Recent academic work in the field

Personal

1. High degree of interest in the growth of the student clinician
2. Respect for the training program where the student is enrolled
3. Willingness to learn and reevaluate opinions regarding educational and therapeutic processes
4. Effective working relationships with teachers and other school personnel
5. Tolerance for differences of opinion
6. Flexibility
7. Patience
8. Sense of humor
9. Willingness to participate in decision making.

RESPONSIBILITIES

Knowledge of the Training Program

To be an effective participant in the training of a student, the master clinician must have knowledge and understanding of the academic and clinical experiences the university provides. This information enables master clinicians to comprehend how student teaching fits into the total training program; for example, no master clinician should expect to feel responsible for the entire training of the student. Knowledge of the background the student brings to the assignment will enable the master clinician to determine the level on which the student should be functioning at the beginning of the assignment. This information answers such questions as, What are the areas of strengths the student already has? and What are the areas that need to be strengthened?

The master clinician should know the criteria and standards established by the university for determining satisfactory completion of the assignment. Knowledge of the expectations of the university faculty enables the master clinician to evaluate with more objectivity the performance of the student clinician.

In the event master clinicians encounter problems, will the university be supportive of them? Master clinicians volunteer an essential service to the training program; therefore, they should receive the full support of the faculty in this endeavor. When the student is a competent clinician, university involvement is minimal; however, when problems are encountered, the master clinician should not be expected to resolve them unilaterally. Problems may range from relatively minor ones to major areas of concern, from inappropriate dress to gross incompetence of a student clinician. Fortunately, most universities have responsible faculty who will respond quickly and appropriately when apprised of problems. There have been instances, however, when the questions and pleas of master clinicians have fallen on deaf ears. Although such situations are frustrating and unfortunate, they are the exception rather than the rule. It is incumbent upon the master clinician to know who makes the final decisions regarding resolution of serious problems. Although a master clinician and university supervisor may have an excellent relationship, the master clinician should know what the university policies are and how supportive and responsive the entire faculty will be in the event problems are encountered.

Requirements of the Assignment

Master clinicians should be knowledgeable of the requirements established by the university regarding the experiences the student clinician is expected to complete. Some training institutions send guidelines to each master clinician describing the requirements of the assignment and specifying the experiences considered of paramount importance in the student's training. (See Appendix for sample guidelines.) Such knowledge gives the master clinician insight into the student's dedication to the assignment. A student may attempt to circumvent some of the requirements, which may indicate a lack of commitment to the assignment. On the other hand, a student may want to participate in more activities than the minimum required. This indicates an interested, highly motivated student.

Frequently all required experiences can be provided on one school site; however, if the assigned school does not house the programs necessary to meet the student teaching requirements, arrangements can be made for some experiences to be acquired on another site. When this is not possible, the university supervisor should be informed of the limitations. Master clinicians may recommend additional experiences, which may be beneficial, such as selected observations and opportunities to work with communication aides. Master clinicians are encouraged to use district resources to supplement university requirements. These additional experiences greatly enhance the student teaching experience and give it an individualized personal touch.

Some training institutions provide students with two assignments, usually a primary (K through 6) site and a secondary (7 through 12) site. Sometimes the second assignment may be a special setting such as a school for the multiply handicapped. When two master clinicians are involved in the training of one student, they must coordinate carefully the two assignments.

It is incumbent upon the master clinician to know the mechanics of the assignments, such as starting date, ending date, number of days per week, hours per day or week, and so forth. This information is necessary if the master clinician is to plan how and when the requirements are to be fulfilled.

Communication Between Master Clinician and University Supervisor

Communication is one of the basic components in a good working relationship. Both the university supervisor and the master clinician should feel free to communicate openly with the other regarding all aspects of the student teaching assignment.

In order to facilitate scheduling and make appropriate arrangements, the master clinicians will need information from the university supervisor regarding the following:

1. The most efficient way and most convenient time to contact the university supervisor

2. Frequency of observations by university supervisor
3. Usual length of visit
4. Method of informing master clinician of observation schedule
5. Special arrangements that may need to be made for the observations
6. Conference arrangements between master clinician and university supervisor, possibly at the conclusion of the observations
7. Evaluation procedures and deadline dates

The master clinician should be prepared to furnish the university supervisor with information, such as the following:

1. How and where master clinician may be contacted, i.e. school or home
2. Procedures for on-site visits
3. Parking arrangements
4. Meeting the principal and other personnel
5. Other information the master clinician believes appropriate to share with the university supervisor

Early resolution of the preceding areas will enable both parties to have a base from which to operate. As in all areas of positive working relationships, good communication gives everyone involved a sense of security. This is particularly helpful in giving the student a sense of cooperation and support for the student teaching experience and assures the master clinician there is a sharing of responsibility.

The First Day

The environment, which is so familiar to the master clinician, is new and strange to the student clinician. Do you remember as a student clinician the first day you took that long walk up the school steps and entered the front door? Or perhaps it was the side door because you could not find the front door from the parking lot. As you looked for the main office, you saw teachers and children scurrying to their rooms. Perhaps you even envied the children; as young as they were, they all knew where they were going and what was expected of them. You were moving down a hall that seemed to have no end! Then came the excitement of being greeted by the speech-language pathologist, your own master clinician, and a new experience had begun!

Master clinicians may remember and should be aware that students have many anxieties about this new and challenging experience. Students have left the sheltered environment of the university to cross over the threshold of academia to the on-the-job environment of the schools. Students look forward to this assignment with mixed emotions. They are eager, fearful, excited, but above all—anxious. During those first days of student teaching, every experience is new. What may be a routine duty for the master clinician can be an anxiety-provoking experience for the student clinician. It must be anticipated that insecurities of the students may be revealed in different ways. Some insecure students give the impression of being very knowledgeable, which may lead master clinicians to assume that students know more than they do; therefore, master clinicians may fail to share necessary basic information with such students. Other students may give the impression that they have been taught nothing, know nothing, and have had no previous exposure to theoretical concepts or clinical procedures. In such situations, master clinicians may spend time reviewing information the student has had and already knows. Fortunately, most students are adequately trained and sufficiently secure that they react and respond in such a way as to portray a realistic picture of their level of competence.

A first day orientation to the new environment diminishes some of the anxieties of student clinicians and helps them over the first day jitters.

Who's Who in the School?

Introducing the student clinician to school personnel informs them that another speech-language pathologist is on site. It is an opportunity to delineate the responsibilities of the student clinician to the personnel and to prepare the way for future contacts. *Hint:* Introducing your assigned student is a subtle way of informing school personnel that you are a respected professional in the field.

What Room? Where?

Knowing your way around the building brings a certain sense of security. It is helpful if student clinicians are shown where the main areas are and how to get there, for instance, the main office, principal's office, nurse's office, cafeteria, teacher's lounge, work room, supply room, and, of course, the therapy room, which may be in an obscure location! It is helpful for student clinicians to have a list of teachers' names, grades, and room numbers.

Where Are You?

There will be occasions when the master clinician or the student clinician must be absent. An exchange of information regarding absences of either one is important in defining areas of responsibilities. Information that should be exchanged includes the following:

A. If master clinician is absent —
  1. Is student to report to school?
  2. If yes, is student to —
    a. conduct therapy?
    b. do observations in classrooms?
    c. work on records?
    d. do other assignments?
B. If student clinician is absent —
  1. Is master clinician to be called at home or school?
  2. Is the school to be notified?
  3. Is there to be a make-up assignment?
  4. If yes, How? When?

Conferences with Student Clinicians

Regularly scheduled conferences give ongoing feedback to the student, which is an important part of the training experience. During the first week or two of the assignment, most master clinicians have found it helpful to establish a set time for conferences. Conferring with the student before the therapy day begins allows the master clinician time to review and critique daily lesson plans prior to their being used. While the student is conducting therapy, the master clinician may write comments to be discussed with the student at a later time. Written comments have proven beneficial, as student clinicians are able to continue therapy without their authority role with the pupils being disrupted. The student can review the comments when it is possible to assimilate the information without the anxieties and pressures of the therapy setting. It has been found helpful to reserve time at the end of the school day when student clinicians may evaluate the day's activities — lesson plans, therapeutic procedures, pupil progress, and, most importantly, their own performance. When appropriate, master clinicians will help students assess their methods for attaining their prescribed objectives and evaluate the pupils' progress. Daily feedback is essential for a student clinician to profit from each day's endeavor.

Evaluation of Student Performance

In few educational experiences do two people spend so much time together as they do in a student teaching assignment. In most instances master clinicians know their student clinicians better than any other person who evaluates the students' professional and clinical competence. Professional and personal assessment is the key to continuing growth in the student teaching assignment, which is an indication of potential growth as a professional. Professional and personal qualities to be evaluated are discussed in Chapter 3.

It is extremely beneficial for master clinicians to apprise students of strengths they are exhibiting. When students are aware of their strengths, they can capitalize on them and use them as the basis for continued development. On the other hand, it is imperative that students be informed of areas of weakness. As areas are identified, students may, through seeking and implementing suggestions, find weaknesses becoming strengths.

When a master clinician identifies areas of weakness to a student and gives suggestions for making improvement, it is anticipated the student will incorporate these suggestions into appropriate professional and personal behaviors. If a student fails to implement suggestions or to find alternative ways to improve performance, it is the responsibility of the master clinician to inform the university supervisor of the student's inability to make appropriate changes.

Sometimes a master clinician feels a student's weaknesses are a reflection of the quality of the master clinician's supervision.

Open communication with the university supervisor can free a master clinician from assuming the entire responsibility of the student's success or failure in the assignment. Master clinicians are sometimes reluctant to state the problems, fearing the student will be disqualified from the field. Usually there are options available to help a weak student, such as additional on-campus practicum, other practicum experiences, additional course work, or independent studies. These options may furnish the student with the background necessary to succeed in the school environment at a later time.

It must be recognized that not every student is a viable candidate for the school setting. Master clinicians must be willing to help the university screen candidates by giving a candid opinion of the eligibility of the student for this environment. When such decisions are to be made, master clinicians should ask themselves, "Would I want this person for a colleague next year?" When the answer is, "Yes," there is no problem. If the answer is, "Not really," then the student has not met the competency requirements of the master clinician. If the answer is, "I don't know," then the master clinician and university supervisor need to analyze carefully the strengths and weaknesses of the student and reach an equitable decision. The competent student is a joy! The borderline student requires extra time and energy. The student who is borderline on-campus and continues as a borderline student clinician in the schools probably will be a borderline speech-language pathologist in the field.

The student who obviously does not meet the competency standards in the student teaching assignment should not be encouraged to continue in the school setting. It is the responsibility of the master clinician to inform the university supervisor, usually in writing, regarding a student's progress in the assignment. When a student is failing, it is the responsibility of the university supervisor to make the decision to withdraw the student or to take the case to the university faculty for suggestions or resolutions. The decision to terminate a student teaching assignment is a traumatic experience for all concerned, but in some situations, it may be necessary.

Some training institutions assign letter grades for student

teaching while others assign Credit/No Credit. Whatever the grading system, the student clinician, the master clinician, and the university supervisor must be aware of the competencies that are expected for satisfactory completion of the assignment. Sufficient information should be supplied by the master clinician so an appropriate grade can be given.

The written evaluation of the student's performance, which the master clinician submits to the university, becomes part of the student's educational placement file. In evaluating a student clinician, the master clinician must keep in mind that a favorable evaluation is a sanction that the student is ready to be hired, perhaps in the same district as the master clinician. The evaluation gives prospective employers a professional opinion of the level of competence the student has attained during the student teaching assignment. Master clinicians must bear in mind that their credibility and judgment are qualities to be valued. It is important that they write this evaluation with professional integrity.

Participation in University Activities

Many university training programs schedule in-service meetings, which are designed to provide information, to clarify procedures, and to exchange opinions relative to the student teaching program. All three sides of the TRIAD may be present—university supervisors, master clinicians, and student clinicians to discuss and evaluate student teaching requirements and their implementation. Or, the master clinicians only may be invited to meet with the faculty. New master clinicians may feel insecure in their role, and this is an opportunity for them to interact in a group of their peers. Whatever the format of the meetings, a dialogue is established within the TRIAD framework, which promotes a more effective system of communication.

Master clinicians may be asked to participate in special campus activities. Often they are invited to speak to university classes concerning therapy techniques and procedures appropriate to the school setting. Master clinicians are sometimes offered part-time faculty appointments to teach beginning courses in the area of their expertise or to supervise in the campus speech and language clinic. Such participation may be a rewarding extension of a master clinician's professional life.

Some universities plan workshops for master clinicians and student clinicians, where selected master clinicians are asked to demonstrate innovative ways in which familiar materials can be used, or they may present materials and techniques they have developed. Both master clinicians and student clinicians leave these workshops with new ideas, which they take back to the school setting. The stimulation of the workshop is that the TRIAD participants share a common experience with a demonstration of *esprit de corps. Hint:* Students appreciate their master clinicians participating in these university planned events.

GUIDELINES

Following are some guidelines to aid master clinicians in supervising students in a successful student teaching assignment.

Screening Procedures

The school setting is unique in that it is the only environment in which hundreds of children spend several hours a day, five days a week, in many different types of activities. Only this setting provides the student clinician with the opportunity to see a myriad of children and to observe the wide range of differences among them. The screening process serves three important functions. The first and foremost function of screening is to aid speech-language pathologists in identifying children who need speech and language remediation. Second, it enables the speech-language pathologist to observe the similarities and differences among normal children. Children share physical, emotional, and intellectual characteristics and behaviors, which develop at particular age levels, but each child basically is unique. Screening is an opportunity for the speech-language pathologist, particularly the student clinician, to observe similarities and differences among children who fall within the broad spectrum of normal. Third, it delineates the accomplishments of the handicapped relative to normal children. When people spend their time with the handicapped, the growth and achievement of the superior performer of that group may be misleading. These children should not be compared to each other but must be evaluated in relation to the performance of normal children. Screening allows speech-language pathologists and student clinicians to maintain an objectivity in assessing the performance of the handicapped child.

The purpose of screening is to identify as efficiently as possible children who need speech and language remediation. Screening helps student clinicians refine their auditory discrimination skills in detecting mild and moderate articulation disorders, language deficits, voice, and rhythm problems. Methods used during screening usually include one or more of the following: articulation tests, repeating words and sentences, and spontaneous speech. Student clinicians need help in learning how to listen and evaluate several features at one time: voice quality, fluency, language development, articulation errors, and appropriateness of response.

Master clinicians should emphasize to student clinicians some general information:

1. Screening must be coordinated with classroom teachers and scheduled so that there will be minimum disruption in classroom activities

2. Screening must be rapid, with as many children as possible being seen in the shortest period of time.

3. Recording of responses must be handled in a concise manner.

Specifically, master clinicians should plan to teach student clinicians the following:

1. How to set up the screening schedule

2. How and when to notify teachers of the screening schedule

3. How to introduce screening procedures to a classroom of pupils

4. How to record and disseminate information collected during screening

5. How to implement procedures for follow-up testing

Selecting a Case Load

One of the most overwhelming experiences in the student assignment is that of selecting the case load. In the campus speech and language clinic, students are usually assigned two or more clients who have already been judged to be in need of therapy and exhibit moderate to severe disorders. It is seldom that the child with a mild problem is referred to a speech-language clinic. In the school setting students are surrounded with a large number of children who exhibit speech and language deviations; therefore, students need guidance in learning the criteria used in case selection.

Although the master clinician is the person who must assume ultimate responsibility for final decisions, students should be encouraged to give opinions with rationale to support their position. Verbalizing their rationale for including or not including children in therapy forces students to organize their thoughts and integrate their theoretical knowledge. Students should also give opinions regarding children who should be grouped together. This participation affords student clinicians a basis for comparison of the similarities and differences between their impressions and the master clinician's decision. Being involved in selecting a case load provides student clinicians with opportunities to think through the selection procedure.

Establishing Therapy Objectives

Student clinicians have learned to develop therapy objectives for their clients in a university speech and language clinic and expect to be involved in this facet of training during student teaching. Most student clinicians may need additional help in writing Individualized Education Programs (Dublinske, 1978). Giving students this responsibility early in the assignment allows them time to practice and perfect this skill.

Both long-term and intermediate objectives of Individualized Education Programs fulfill a purpose that is different from that of traditional lesson plans. These objectives cover weeks, months, and even a year, while lesson plans are specific to each day's therapy session.

Lesson Plans

Daily lesson plans are the bane of existence for most student clinicians. Often master clinicians are reluctant to require daily lesson plans from student clinicians; however, experience has shown there is value in having students discipline themselves to write them. Although students complain about writing lesson plans, it is not the writing itself that is difficult or time-consuming. The difficulty lies in the tedious planning that is required to insure a successful therapy session.

A careful review of lesson plans by the master clinician over a period of time is an aid in identifying strengths and weaknesses of the student clinician. Some signs of weaknesses that may be identified are that the student is not prepared, is overly dependent on materials, is not providing enough activities to attain the goals of the therapy session, is not planning daily objectives that move toward the intermediate goals, and is rigid and unable to deviate from the planned lesson when the situation warrants modification. Areas of strengths that can be observed through use of lesson plans are that the student is organized, is well prepared, demonstrates a sense of direction, exhibits a sense of continuity in lesson planning, shows ability to build on previous lessons, meets the needs of the individual child and the group, and is flexible and sufficiently secure so appropriate on-the-spot modifications can be made.

Lesson plans with written comments from master clinicians to student clinicians are valuable references for students to use in the future. Students will find it helpful to review critical comments of performance and methods used. They are records of techniques used with pupils presenting different disorders, appropriateness of methods and techniques employed, and the response of pupils to these various methods and techniques. *Suggestion:* If the master clinician makes a carbon copy of these written comments, this precludes misunderstandings that could arise at a later time.

Some master clinicians have students fold a page into four

sections and write a lesson plan in each section. This gives the student clinician and the master clinician a quick assessment of the continuity of ongoing therapy. On the reverse side of the page, student clinicians write their evaluations of the completed session. The lesson may have been beautiful in theory, but the kids were bored, the activity overrode the value of the objective, the clinician did all the talking. Self-evaluation plays an integral role in assessing the effectiveness of therapy and contributes to the professional growth of the clinician.

Individual/Group Therapy

Before beginning their assignments in the school setting, most students have accumulated a considerable number of practicum hours in the campus speech and language clinic. In most instances these clinical hours have been with clients in individual sessions. Although such experiences are extremely valuable and aid clinicians in forming a solid base for remediation techniques, most student clinicians have had little or no experience with *group* therapy. Many will have had group management techniques in theory, but they need to develop the skills of working with groups of children during their student teaching assignment.

Student clinicians who have not had previous group experience need help in developing lessons for each child within the group and guidance in implementing them. Effective group dynamics take place when student clinicians have learned how to incorporate the needs of each child into a group therapy session and to use peer interaction to achieve remedial goals. The activity chosen must meet the needs of each individual as well as the group as a whole. Careful planning allows the student clinician to focus on the group goal and the objectives for each child. Leonard (1976) suggested the following ways to help student clinicians learn group techniques:

1. Have students set up groups with master clinicians (don't do it for them); be sure student clinicians have a rationale for grouping children together.
2. Try a sociogram and ask students to study group dynamics and interactions.

3. Have student clinicians try different physical arrangements with their groups.
4. Have student clinicians observe master clinician; have some lessons shared as team effort.
5. Discuss types of appropriate activities; experiment and have student clinicians evaluate success/failure.
6. Have student clinicians tape a session, listen to it, and analyze it.
7. Be aware this aspect of speech-language therapy is a new experience for most student clinicians. *Caution:* go slowly, do not expect student clinicians automatically to be able to handle all areas of group sessions.

Beginning Therapy

Master clinicians are not in agreement when student clinicians should begin conducting therapy. Representing differing positions, the following comments are made frequently by master clinicians: "I allow student clinicians to observe me until they feel ready, and then I ease them into handling the case load," and "I don't want a carbon copy of myself, so I present them with my case load when they first begin their assignment."

The problem with the first approach is that weak students may feel they are not ready to begin therapy until the assignment is half over. The result is insufficient time for suggestions to be incorporated, for growth to take place, for a competent level of performance to be attained, and for performance to be evaluated. The obvious problem with the second method is that the student is plunged into a new experience with shocking suddenness to sink or swim. That so many swim is a credit to native ability for survival and to the training received at the university.

Skilled master clinicians have a sense for the student orientation period. Experience has shown that some observation of the master clinician is helpful to the beginning student clinician. A suggested guideline is for a student to observe approximately three times and then ease into the case load by selecting one pupil or one group of pupils and to assume responsibility for all the pupils in the case load by the fifth week.

Terminating Therapy

Many student clinicians have had limited experience in participating in the dismissal of pupils from therapy. The reasons for student participation in the dismissal process of therapy is similar to the rationale for student participation in the selection of pupils as previously discussed in the section Selecting a Case Load. Participation by student clinicians in testing, decision making, and final report writing for termination of therapy is an important part of student teaching. Master clinicians should impart to the student clinician the policy of the district as well as their own judgment for termination of speech and language cases. It is important for students to have a basic point of reference that they can use to compare their judgments with an experienced professional. Students learn and grow professionally by exposure to proven methods, procedures, and rationale.

Sharing Materials

To share or not to share. That is a question many new master clinicians ask. Some master clinicians willingly share their materials and encourage their student clinicians to dip freely into the treasure chest, whereas others expect student clinicians to develop their own supply of materials. Both opinions have merit. To encourage student clinicians to be inventive and creative challenges them to seek out and develop materials on their own. On the other hand, some materials that master clinicians have accumulated are special, rare, or expensive, and it is a generous gesture to allow student clinicians to use these valued materials.

Budgets

Frequently speech-language pathologists find they need skills in planning a budget. It is important to know how to plan, select, and price materials and equipment. When speech-language pathologists go into a setting where they are expected to purchase materials and equipment or set up a language learning center, it is necessary to understand the process of budgeting in order to make appropriate decisions. Some master clinicians have devised hypothetical situations for their student clinicians, such as having them select materials and estimate the cost of equiping a language learning center. Such exercises give student clinicians a comprehensive picture of how to set up a program and how much it will cost.

Working with Communication Aides

Master clinicians who have communication aides should orient student clinicians to working with paraprofessionals. Learning to organize one's own time with efficiency and dispatch is difficult, but it may become an awesome task when someone else is to be guided through the daily activities. Student clinicians should be aware of the additional responsibility involved in training and directing communication aides. Master clinicians can give student clinicians experience by having them organize the aide's work load and stating in written form what is expected of the aide. Together master clinician and student clinician can evaluate the effectiveness of the work performed by the aide. Learning how to work effectively with communication aides is an important part of training of a student clinician.

Establishing Effective Relationships with School Personnel

Governments may legislate, states may mandate, and districts may demand, but the speech-language pathologist is the one who brings the speech and language program to fulfillment. Establishing effective relationships with school and community personnel is vital to the success of the speech and language program. Incoming student clinicians may feel overwhelmed by the number of people with whom they have contact in the school program. *Hint:* Giving a list of names of school personnel and their duties is helpful to the student clinician.

Some student clinicians need to be encouraged to become acquainted with classroom teachers. Learning to socialize in the casual environment of morning break allows for professional exchanges to evolve later. It should be emphasized to student clinicians that professionalism is not limited to the therapy room environment; a cheerful outlook, promptness in handling communication, and consideration of the feelings of others are part of every job success.

Meeting with Parents and Other Professionals

One of the learning experiences student clinicians will have by participating in Individualized Education Programs is observing the variation of parental responses: overly concerned, irate, hostile, cooperative, as well as the hard-to-contact and the no-shows. Although many students have had some experience in conferring with parents in the campus speech-language clinic, their involvement in Individualized Education Program conferences in the school setting provides student clinicians an additional opportunity to learn by doing. Novice speech-language clinicians often find it difficult to use simple, direct language when communicating with parents. Sometimes students find it hard to be specific when giving information to teachers and other school personnel. Participation in the Individualized Education Program conferences affords students the opportunity to develop an effective, flexible approach. There are occasions when student clinicians could participate in special school functions, such as faculty meetings and P.T.A. meetings. Encouraging students to discuss the speech-language program at such meetings helps them develop poise and self-confidence.

Record Keeping

Paperwork! Paperwork! No job is finished until the paperwork is done! A contributing factor to job fatigue is coping with the increasing amount of paperwork. *Helpful hint:* Let student clinicians participate in record keeping and report writing. Learning to organize time to include daily progress reports, anecdotal records, pupil attendance, conference reports, and so forth is all part of being a competent school speech-language pathologist.

The preceding discussion is intended to serve as a guide in several of the areas that have been of concern to master clinicians. The guidelines presented previously are not meant to be all-inclusive. Creative master clinicians will expand the list to include areas unique to their situations.

CONCLUSION

Master clinicians have an opportunity to exert a significant influence on student clinicians. Students enter the school setting at a time in their professional training when they are emerging from the academic environment and moving into the work setting. During this period, master clinicians are guiding and molding impressionable novice clinicians. Master clinicians must realize their influence will make a lasting impression during this formative period in the students' professional training. In some ways this experience is as critical as two or three years in the academic environment.

Although it is a demanding responsibility to be a master clinician when the eyes of both the university training program and the student clinician are focused on the effort put forth by master clinicians, it is hoped they find their role and contribution exciting and rewarding. The conscientious effort of master clinicians in helping to train students deserves a big thank you from the other members of the TRIAD.

Chapter 7

SPEECH–LANGUAGE SERVICES IN COMMUNITY COLLEGES

COMMUNITY COLLEGE AS A SETTING

The community college is the newest professional opportunity for speech-language pathologists. Special education programs at this academic level have expanded during the past few years, bringing new challenges and opportunities to those interested in working with adults who have communication disorders. This chapter will discuss the community college as an employment setting for speech-language pathologists in an academic-occupational setting with individuals over eighteen years of age.

Traditionally, community colleges have offered an academic objective of an associate of arts degree. Upon completion of this degree, students made one of two decisions: to terminate their formal education after the fourteenth year or to transfer to a four-year college to earn a bachelor of arts/science degree. In recent years, however, academic objectives have expanded to encompass occupational education, vocational training, and continuing education.

Formerly, the terms junior college and city college were used for two-year academic institutions. In recent years the more inclusive title community college has been used. This change in title reflects the changing philosophy of the two-year college. According to Bailey, the community college is becoming one of the educational centers of creative and experimental leadership (1975).

As the term implies, community colleges are locally based. A community college, as an institution of higher learning, is obliged to be responsive to the educational needs of those who live within its geographic borders. The student population is varied in interests, background, and age. The community college system gives evidence that higher education is no longer just for the young, it

113

is becoming an educational site for all ages and interests. Course offerings reflect a wide range of academic, vocational, and avocational pursuits. Community college catalogs list a variety of educational experiences, such as conversational Chinese, survey of psychology, calculus, speaking English as a second language, auto mechanics, computer science, upholstering, cosmetology, and manual communication skills. Courses reflect the background and interest of the students, and classes are scheduled to meet the diverse needs of this student population.

Individuals in community colleges may choose one or more of the following educational options:

1. Earn an associate of arts degree
2. Complete course work to meet lower division requirements of four-year colleges
3. Pursue occupational education and attain appropriate certification
4. Attend continuing education classes: lecture series, workshops, and so forth for credit or noncredit

The community college offers opportunities and advantages, which make it attractive as a center of learning:

1. As a local institution of higher education, it is responsive to the community it serves.
2. Classes generally are smaller than many universities, which allows for more personalized attention.
3. Students with subject or grade deficiencies precluding their acceptance to a four-year college have opportunities to correct these deficiencies at the community college.
4. Community colleges are less expensive than their four-year counterparts:
   a. Students can live at home.
   b. Travel expenses are minimal.
   c. Tuition and fees are low.
5. The Selected High School Student Program enables students currently enrolled in secondary schools to apply community college courses toward high school graduation.
6. Students with foreign language backgrounds find courses in English organized specifically for their needs.

"The community college also recognizes that one of its prime purposes is to offer opportunities for individuals to continue through their lives the process of actualizing their human potentials and enhancing their sense of self-esteem while learning life skills" (Breakey et al., 1978, p. 3). One community college states its philosophy: a two-year college is "a community oriented institution committed to providing general and specialized educational opportunities for all individuals regardless of race, nationality, creed, age, sex or physical disability. . . [the] primary purpose is to provide an atmosphere where individuals are stimulated to further their intellectual, social and personal development so that they can become productive and effective citizens" (Pasadena Area Community College District, 1980, p. 1).

An increase in numbers and types of students who are enrolling in public and private community colleges has been observed by Bailey (1975). A contributing factor is that federal legislation mandates special education for the handicapped from three through twenty-one years if federal funds are used by the educational institution. Passage of federal and state legislation for the handicapped has increased the demand for services for all types of disabilities: learning disabled, physically disabled, blind, deaf, hearing impaired, and communicatively disabled. To meet the needs of handicapped individuals, community colleges are expanding their special education services to enable all students to benefit from the curricula.

An increasing number of learning disabled individuals are now reentering the educational system. Some have been dropouts whose inability to cope successfully with academics forced them to leave school at early ages. Others have been in special education classes and are advised by high school counselors to seek educational opportunities at the community college. The number of physically handicapped individuals attending college also is increasing. Existing and new buildings are being constructed to accommodate them, and advanced technology is enabling many of them to enjoy greater mobility.

The number of deaf and hearing impaired students usually is dependent upon the quality of the special services offered. Interpreters, tutors, and specialized counselors increase attendance of this population. Community colleges with high quality services are an attraction for the deaf and hearing impaired to attend that particular institution.

Speech-Language Population

The population served by the speech-language pathologist is drawn from the total community college and includes students whose disability is in speech-language-hearing only while some have additional disabilities. They evidence the variety of problems found at the high school level or at other clinical settings. In community colleges there may be young adults who have sustained head injuries and, after sufficient recovery, are returning to school to prepare themselves for career or vocational pursuits.

Many students who come for speech-language services have had previous help in school, clinics, hospitals, or other facilities. These students often are at a turning point in their lives; the alleviation of their communication disorder is important for their career or vocational goals. The hearing impaired may need continued monitoring in order to maintain adequate communication skills. There may be some students who have never had the opportunity for speech-language services; they may come from remote areas, from foreign countries, or their problem is of recent origin.

Only a few studies have been conducted to quantify the population in need of speech-language-hearing services and the status of such services in community colleges. A study conducted by Smith et al. (1976) revealed that 3.0 percent of the college population had articulation disorders, 0.99 percent voice disorders, 1.88 percent stuttering problems, 0.28 percent language disorders, and an additional 0.88 percent had multiple speech-language disorders. Hearing impairments were not included in this data. To be counted in this particular investigation, the disorder had to be severe enough to preclude free choice of profession on the part of the randomly selected students. The results of this study would indicate that a little over 6 percent of the community college enrollment have communication disorders due to speech-language problems, which impede development of their full potential as free choosing individuals. In other studies the percentage of students with communication disorders ranged from 4 percent to 10 percent (Breakey et al, 1978; Gottlieb, 1967).

A study was conducted by Breakey et al. (1977) in which a questionnaire was sent to ninety-three California community colleges. Of the forty-four respondents, twenty community colleges provided some speech-language-hearing services with a speech-language pathologist employed on a full– or part-time basis. It is interesting to note that most of these speech-language pathologists were assigned both clinical and academic duties. Academic duties included teaching courses in normal language development, voice and diction, story telling, child development, introduction to communication disorders, introduction to exceptional children, and English as a second language.

To determine the status of speech-language-hearing services in community colleges on the east coast, a study was conducted in New York, New Jersey, and Connecticut (Chapey et al., 1977). Information was sought regarding screening, evaluation, remediation, instruction in speech or language improvement, and instruction for bilingual students. Of the colleges 66 percent responded, and the results indicated that 62 percent offered at least one service. A little less than one-half of the respondents offered speech improvement, and approximately one-third offered instruction to bilingual students. Few community colleges offered screening, evaluation, or remediation services in speech and hearing.

In a survey of the twenty-eight publicly supported community colleges in Florida (Peters, 1980), it was found that approximately five provided some speech-language-hearing services, such as hearing evaluations, clinical speech-language services, and speech for foreign students. The majority of the five colleges employ speech-language pathologists on a part-time basis and provide limited services. Miami-Dade Community College, which offers comprehensive services, describes its clinical program as follows: "Language, speech and hearing disorder services are available . . . These services include diagnosis, prognosis and treatment of all types of language, speech and hearing disorders. Therapy is conducted on an individual/group basis by Certified Communication Disorder Specialists. The clinics are modern and well equipped. Efforts are made to match appointments with students' schedules" (1979–81 catalog, p. 35). Several of the colleges offer a course called "Introduction to Speech-Language Pathology/Disorders." One college, Broward Community College, has an additional course, "Introduction to Audiology."

As stated earlier, 4 to 10 percent of the community college population have communication disorders; however, the preceding studies have shown only a small percentage of the colleges provide ample services for these individuals. With the implementation of federal legislation, the Rehabilitation Act of 1973, speech-language-hearing services in community colleges should be expanding. Some community colleges have developed or are in the process of developing model programs. It is anticipated that administrators of other community colleges will recognize the need and support more comprehensive services for the communicatively handicapped. Services should be designed to aid communicatively disabled individuals achieve maximum interaction within the college by providing assessment, educational, and/or therapeutic services and other necessary assistance.

IMPLEMENTATION OF THE PROGRAM

Some speech-language pathologists may find they are hired to develop a speech and language program, while others are hired to work in an established ongoing program. This section will discuss implementation of a program for the speech-language pathologist who is new to this setting.

Speech-Language Pathologist

Qualifications

Qualifications for employment at the community college level vary from state to state. In some cases certification requirements are established by the local community college districts, while in other states certification requirements are established by state boards of education or other agencies. To maintain a quality program, the speech-language pathologist should hold a master's degree in speech-language pathology. It is recommended that the speech-language pathologist also hold state licensing in those states which issue licenses. Certification of Clinical Competence in Speech-Language Pathology from the American Speech-Language-Hearing Association is highly desirable, especially if student clinicians from university programs are to receive supervised clinical training at the community college.

Qualities deemed necessary for a speech-language pathologist in the community college are as follows:

1. Shows high degree of interest in the field of speech-language-hearing
2. Keeps abreast of new information, techniques, materials, and equipment for the communicatively handicapped
3. Has background experience working with young and mature adults
4. Is flexible in methods and techniques
5. Relates well to various age and interest groups
6. Is a problem solver (many programs at community colleges are in their infancy, and speech-language pathologists may be developing and establishing new speech-language programs)
7. Works well with administrators, faculty, and community
8. Has supervisory expertise (many speech-language pathologists are in charge of tutors, aides, secretaries, and so on)
9. Has an understanding of managing budgets
10. Takes initiative and follows through

The speech-language pathologist must maintain a demeanor that assures respect and confidence from the student and must maintain an objectivity about the student and the communication problem. The speech-language pathologist must project an attitude that is encouraging, realistic, and personally meaningful to the student. At this level it may be easy for the speech-language pathologist to become a friend or peer; however, this interferes with maintaining objectivity and a professional attitude between student and speech-language pathologist.

Duties and Responsibilities

Duties and responsibilities vary depending upon such factors as size of college, size of speech-language program, and types of services offered.

There are few written guidelines for speech-language pathologists in community colleges. Many speech-language pathologists have been concerned about the absence of guidelines for this level of education, and in 1976, the Consortium of California Community College Speech-Language-Hearing Programs was established. Duties and responsibilities of the speech-language pathologist developed by the consortium are included here.

I. The Speech/Language and Hearing Therapist should have responsibilities for determining and utilizing appropriate procedures for identification, diagnosis, referral, caseload, selection, case termination, and follow-up, which includes:

   1. Employment of reliable assessment procedures, techniques, and standardized tests necessary for thorough and accurate diagnosis and assessment of pupil needs and behavior.
   2. Formulation of short and long-term intervention goals and objectives to meet individual needs.
   3. Redefinition of objectives and modifications of habilitation and instructional procedures as needed.
   4. Utilization of research strategies and results to improve program and case management.
   5. Establishment of effective working relationships with school personnel and other professionals.
   6. Cooperation with local district, community, regional, state, and federal programs to effect comprehensive services, research, and/or training of personnel.

II. Speech/Language and Hearing Therapist, using ongoing assessment and evaluation procedures, should establish general and specific pupil instructional objectives which include:

   1. Realistic concept of the prognosis and ultimate goals clients can be expected to achieve.
   2. Establishment of communication skill objectives which reflect the client's abilities as well as the limitations imposed by restricting factors revealed in assessment.
   3. Written goals, and objectives, in the therapy plan for each client which are consonant with the goals and objectives of the client's total educational program.
   4. Systematic review of diagnostic findings, instructional and clinical methods, and client progress.

5. Maintenance of daily records of performance.
6. Securing additional evaluations and/or professional consultation when the client fails to make satisfactory progress.

III. Program Management responsibilities for the supervisor should include:

1. Development of a list of needs, goals, and measurable objectives for the program.
2. Establishment of program guidelines and procedures for screening, scheduling, referral, case selection, and case termination.
3. Formulation of a formal data collection system for program and case management and for local, state, and national reports, and for evaluation of the total language, speech and hearing program.
4. Preparation and dissemination of information about speech/language and hearing services to school personnel, public and private agencies, the community, and the profession.
5. Coordination with school and other public and private agencies in making and accepting referrals following formal procedures. To provide comprehensive services for communicatively handicapped students.
6. Applying results of research in continuing program development and evaluation and encouraging and coordinating research projects.
7. Preparation of program requests and budgets.
8. Ordering and maintenance of equipment, supplies and materials.
9. Providing systematic student observation and practical experience in cooperation with colleges and universities.
10. Assisting in recruitment, interviewing applicants and making recommendations for employment and dismissal of professional and para-professional staff.
11. Encouragement and development of professional interests, talents, and leadership potential of individual clients and staff.
12. Developing school and community programs to increase

awareness of speech/language and hearing problems.

13. Providing clients with information and assistance.
14. Developing in-service training for staff, communication aides, administrators, and other school personnel.
15. Formulating and writing program and grant proposals.
16. Serving as a resource person in assisting staff with complex diagnostic and remedial cases.*

In addition to the foregoing duties and responsibilities, most speech-language pathologists will find it advantageous to be active in their state associations as well as in organizations for the handicapped. Community college speech-language services are being shaped by those who are currently developing programs; therefore, it is beneficial to be an active participant in groups and associations engaged in these endeavors.

Delivery of Services

A speech-language-hearing pathology program is designed to deliver clinical services to adults within the college who have a communicative disability. The purpose of the program is to assist these students to develop communication skills that are essential for effective interaction on campus, at work, and in the community. The program's goals should be to provide direct, intensive, and individualized clinical services to effect positive changes in communicative behavior and to provide information and assistance to the other programs on campus (Community Colleges Chancellor's Office, in press).

To develop and implement a good clinical program requires initiative and purpose. To maintain an effective clinical program requires a steadfastness of purpose and an awareness of those qualities which will influence productivity and growth of the program. Most speech-language pathologists desire to create an innovative program as well as one that is built on a solid foundation. Sometimes it is difficult to keep all parts of the program

---

*From L. Breakey, S. Kesterson, B. Price, and L. Rasmussen, Community Colleges and the Speech Pathologist. California Speech and Hearing Association ad hoc Committee Report Presented at California Speech and Hearing Association Annual Convention, March 27, 1977, San Francisco, California.

running smoothly in a coordinated effort. Basic procedures are necessary for all clinical programs; however, the implementation of these procedures are unique to each setting. Following is a list of procedures and a discussion of ways to implement them in a community college setting:

1. Identifying the need
2. Identifying referral sources
3. Assessment procedures
4. Case selection
5. Scheduling students for therapy
6. Writing Individualized Education Programs for students scheduled for therapy
7. Materials and equipment
8. Professional relations
9. Use of communication aides

Identifying the Need

One question that must be answered is the extent of the *need* for the speech-language-hearing service. It has been stated previously that 4 to 10 percent of the community college population have a need for speech and language therapy; however, this figure does not represent a particular community. The needs of the community can be estimated by contacting both campus and community sources. On-campus sources are faculty, health services, counseling centers, other special education programs, and students. Community sources that can be contacted are feeder high schools, departments of rehabilitation, hospitals, social welfare offices, community organizations, speech-language-hearing clinics, and so forth.

Of prime importance is letting students know that services are offered on campus and where these services are housed. There are several ways this can be accomplished. A write-up in the college newspaper using an interview format and picture of the new faculty member gains recognition of the program by the students. A bulletin announcing speech-language-hearing services and procedures for making an appointment can be posted where students congregate. Contacting counselors and familiarizing them with the program will enable them to give information to students in need of these services. Speech-language clinic services should be listed in the schedule of classes and described in the college catalog.

Identifying Referral Sources

Referrals are generally from three sources:

SELF-REFERRAL. In some speech-language programs, there is a form that is filled out by students during registration, thus identifying their need for speech-language-hearing services. At this level students usually are eager to avail themselves of the special services offered on campus; therefore, they often refer themselves once they know a speech-language pathologist is available.

CAMPUS. Sources for on-campus referrals are counseling centers, psychology services, handicapped programs, remedial reading programs, learning resource centers, health services, departments of speech communication, drama, telecommunication, broadcasting, and English as a second language program.

OFF-CAMPUS AGENCIES. Some community referral sources are state departments of rehabilitation, private speech-language-hearing clinics, hospital rehabilitation departments, feeder high schools, private medical practitioners, and university speech-language-hearing clinics.

Making oneself and one's program known to college information personnel helps students receive assistance in finding the office of the speech-language pathologist.

Assessment Procedures

The first appointment the student schedules with the speech-language pathologist is a screening assessment. Subsequent appointments provide the speech-language pathologist with more definitive information. When the initial appointment is made, it is helpful to have students fill out a short intake form (see Appendix). This provides the speech-language pathologist with pertinent information when interviewing students and assessing their speech-language problems, and it provides a record of those who have inquired about speech-language services. After the initial interview, an appointment is made for a more thorough assessment. Based on the results of the assessment, an Individualized Education Program is written.

"If it is determined that the needs of the student cannot be met by the speech-language-hearing program, it is the responsibility of the communicative disability specialist to refer the student to another agency, either on campus or in the community, which can more effectively deal with the problem" (Community Colleges Chancellor's Office, in press).

Case Selection

The population served by the speech-language pathologist should be drawn from the total college program, both day and evening enrollment. Generally, the criteria for enrollment in the program are as follows:

1. The student must be a resident of the community college district or an interdistrict transfer.
2. The student must be enrolled in the college.
3. The student, in some colleges, is required to carry a specified number of units to be eligible for speech-language services.
4. The student must have a speech-language disability that presents limitations educationally, occupationally, and/or socially.

Further criteria are that assessment results must indicate that speech-language-hearing services can be of potential value and the student indicates his willingness to meet the requirements agreed upon between himself and the speech-language pathologist, for example, the student must be responsible for attendance, notification when absent, and completion of outside assignments. Being able to coordinate speech-language personnel with the student's schedule is another factor influencing enrollment.

Scheduling Students for Therapy

The way students are enrolled into the speech-language program depends upon the procedure that has been established within each community college. In many programs students register for a class titled "Speech Clinic." Usually a specified number of units are given for students who enroll and fulfill the requirements, such as weekly or semiweekly attendance in clinic, additional hours with a communication aide, and/or required outside assignments. In most community college programs, grading is credit/no credit. In order to fulfill course requirements, students are expected to attend regularly and spend outside time on remedial techniques recommended by the speech-language pathologist.

Some students may have difficulty with the additional responsibility of therapy. Many students at the community college level are enrolled in heavy academic schedules and are working part or full time. This added responsibility may aid students in establishing their priorities.

At this educational level, students are usually committed to coming regularly for therapy. To insure attendance and punctuality, the speech-language pathologist should inform the student of his obligation to the therapeutic arrangements. When students are given a schedule and room assignment, they also should be given the clinic telephone number and told to call if they must cancel an appointment. It is advisable to inform students that if they miss appointments without good reason, they will be dropped from therapy. Experience has shown that most students desire help, and they are on time and attend regularly.

If students are to be dropped from therapy because of absenteeism or not following through on assignments, they should be told of this decision in person, by phone, or by letter. It is wise to leave the option available for speech-language help in the future. When students are not ready to effect the changes necessary to correct a communication disorder, it can be an insightful experience for them when they realize this for themselves. Sometimes a suggestion for services from other facilities, such as a community speech and language center or private clinic, may be appropriate. When students understand the expense of speech-language services outside the educational setting, they usually put greater effort into therapy.

Considering that 4 to 10 percent of the community college population is in need of speech-language-hearing services, it readily can be seen that an effective program must be designed to offer service to a large number of students. One effective means, when possible, is to group students in therapy. This can be done when facilities are large enough to accommodate several students and their needs can be met in a group setting. Increased speech-language services may be attained by use of communication aides, who have been trained and are supervised by the speech-language pathologist. Communication aides may be volunteers, or they may be paid through various funding sources, such as work study programs, or in the case of interpreters, they are paid from state funds allocated for the deaf and hearing impaired population.

Some speech-language pathologists set aside several hours a week for special appointments. This provides them with a stated time to see referrals and schedule students for additional therapy as needed.

Individualized Education Programs

One difference between secondary and community college students is their approach to therapy. The secondary pupil is often finding himself, is unsure of his goals, and is concerned about his developing self-image, whereas the community college student may be characterized as being goal oriented. At this age most students have definite goals in mind and approach speech-language therapy as a means of achieving them, for example, a student may present himself because of a distorted /s/. When it is learned his career goal is to become an actor, the decision to remediate the articulation problem is of immediate importance for the student and the speech-language pathologist. The mature student may be involved actively in writing his Individualized Education Program as a means of capitalizing on his initial motivation and using his participation as a base for continued motivation. Therapy can follow the interests expressed by the student with material slanted toward his goals and interests. At times it may be advisable to involve other specialists from the handicapped programs to maximize the services offered a student. From time to time revision of the Individualized Education Program may be necessary for the student's highest potential to be achieved. Therapy should be terminated when the communication potential is reached or there is no further demonstrable progress. Should the latter occur, the perceptive speech-language pathologist seeks other referrals for the student. An important function of therapy is to help the student realize what can and cannot be accomplished in speech-language therapy.

Materials and Equipment

A variety of materials and equipment is necessary to work effectively with the wide range of disorders and ages of students in community colleges. Following is a list of materials and equipment deemed appropriate for working with communicatively handicapped students at this level.

ASSESSMENT INSTRUMENTS

Austin Spanish Articulation Test, Learning Concepts, 2501 N. Lamar, Austin, TX 78705.

Boehm Test of Basic Concepts, Boehm, A., Psychological Corp., 304 E. 45th St., New York, NY 10017.

Clinical Evaluation of Language Functions, Charles Merrill, Publ. Co., 1300 Alum Creek Dr., Columbus, OH 43216.

Detroit Test of Language Learning Ability, The Bobbs-Merrill Co. Inc., 4500 W. 62nd St., Indianapolis, IN 46206.

Goldman-Fristoe Test of Articulation, American Guidance Service, Inc., Publishers' Building, Circle Pines, MN 55014.

Goldman-Fristoe-Woodcock Auditory Skills Test Battery, American Guidance Service, Inc., Publishers' Building, Circle Pines, MN 55014.

Illinois Test of Psycholinguistic Ability, Kirk, S., McCarthy, J. and Kirk, W., Western Psychological Services, 12031 Wilshire Blvd., Los Angeles, CA 90025.

Jeffers-Barley Lipreading Test, Speech Reading (Lipreading), Charles C Thomas, Publ., 2600 South First Street, Springfield, IL 62717.

Language Samples: written and oral

Lindamood Test of Auditory Conceptualization, Lindamood, C. and Lindamood, P., Teaching Resources, 100 Boylston St., Boston, MA 02116.

Minnesota Test for Differential Diagnosis of Aphasia, Schuell, H., University of Minnesota Press, Minneapolis, MN.

Northwestern Syntax Sentence Test, Lee, L., Northwestern University Press, Chicago, IL.

Peabody Picture Vocabulary Test (Revised), American Guidance Service, Inc. Publishers' Building, Circle Pines, MN 55014.

Porch Index of Communicative Ability, Porch, B., Consulting Psychologists Press, 577 College Ave., Palo Alto, CA 94306.

Programmed Therapy for Stuttering in Children and Adults, Ryan, B., Charles C Thomas, Publ., 2600 South First Street, Springfield, IL 62717.

Quick Neurological Screening, Academic Therapy Publications, Inc., 20 Commercial Blvd., Novato, CA 94947.

Templin-Darley Articulation Test, Bureau of Educational Research and Service, Extension Division, State University of Iowa, Iowa City, IA 52240.

Test of Auditory Comprehension of Language, (TACL), Learning Concepts, 2301 N. Lamar, Austin, TX 78705.

Test of Auditory Discrimination, (TAD), Academic Therapy Publications, Inc., 20 Commercial Blvd., Novato, CA 94747.

Token Test, de Renzi, E. and Vignolo, L.: Test for aphasics. *Brain, 85:*665–678, 1962.

Wepman Auditory Discrimination Test, Wepman, J., Western Psychological Services, 12031 Wilshire Blvd., Los Angeles, CA 90025.

Wilson Voice Profile, Wilson, D., *Voice Problems of Children,* The Williams & Wilkins Co., 428 Preston St., Baltimore, MD 21202.

Woodcock-Johnson Psycho-Educational Battery, (language section), Teaching Resources, 100 Boylston St., Boston, MA 02116.

COMMERCIAL THERAPY MATERIALS

Bush, C., *Language Remediation and Expansion,* Communication Skill Builders, Inc., 815 E. Broadway, Tucson, AZ 85733.

Engelmann, S. and Osborn, J., *Distar Language III,* Science Research Assoc., Inc., 155 N. Wacker Dr., Chicago, IL 60606.

Fairbanks, G., *Voice and Articulation Drillbook,* Harper & Row, Publ., Inc., 10 E. 53rd St., New York, NY 10022.

Fisher, H. *Improving Voice and Articulation,* Houghton-Mifflin Co., 2 Park St., Boston, MA 02107.

Fokes, J., *Fokes Sentence Builder,* Teaching Resources, 100 Boylston St., Boston, MA 02116.

Herr, S., *Developing Auditory Awareness and Insight,* Instructional Materials & Equipment Distributors, 1520 Cotner Ave., Los Angeles, CA 90025.

Keirsey, D. and Bates, M., *Please Understand Me,* Prometheus Nemesis Books, 131 21st St., Del Mar, CA 92014.

Lindamood, C. and Lindamood, P., *Auditory Discrimination In Depth,* Teaching Resources Corp., 100 Boylston Ave., Boston, MA 02116.

Los Angeles Unified School District, *Bridging the Asian Language and Cultural Gap,* Modulearn, Inc., 32158 Camino Capistrano, San Juan Capistrano, CA 92675.

Luter, J., *Speech Sounds in Action*, Burgess Publ. Co., 7108 Ohms Lane, Minneapolis, MN 55435.

McKee, B., *Phonemic Approximation: Workbooks for /r/, /s/, /l/. /ch/*, Bob McKee, 3415 Ione, Los Angeles, CA 90068.

Medlin, V. and Warnock, H., *Basic Set of Word Making Cards*, Word Making Productions, 70 W. Louise Ave., Salt Lake City, UT 84115.

PEP: Auditory Perceptual Enhancement Program, Modern Education Corp., P.O. Box 721, Tulsa, OK 74101.

Schaffer, F., *Frank Schaffer Publications: Understanding What you Read; Drawing Conclusions; Prefixes, Suffixes and Syllabication; Antonyms, Synonyms and Homonyms* (workbooks), Teaching Aid Specialties, 245 Bloom Dr., Monterey Park, CA 91754.

Speech Illustrated Cards, Stryker Illustrations, 1674 Meridian Ave., Suite 201, Miami Beach, FL 33139.

Travis Story Pictures, Lee Travis, 3412 Red Rose Dr., Encino, CA 91436.

MISCELLANEOUS THERAPY MATERIALS

Dictionary

Newspaper articles

Reader's Digest

Scripts — two-person dialogues

    Theatrical

    Television

    Radio

Thesaurus

World Atlas

EQUIPMENT

Phonic Mirrors®

Tape recorders, including small cassette recorders for student use

Video recorder and monitors, often available from telecommunication departments or from audiovisual instructional aid centers

Delayed auditory feedback

Language Masters®

Tokbaks®

Auditory trainers

The preceding are suggested assessment instruments, therapy materials, and equipment, and they are not intended to cover all the excellent materials available.

Professional Relations

To further the goals of the program, the successful speech-language pathologist exerts every effort to develop satisfactory professional relationships. Maintaining a dynamic and cooperative relationship with other campus and community programs is important. Some programs have failed to reach their potential because the speech-language pathologist was unable to work cooperatively with others. To develop and maintain a strong program, the support of the following personnel and programs is recommended: (1) deans, (2) counselors, (3) handicapped service personnel, (4) occupation and career departments, (5) departments of English and speech, (6) English as a second language program, (7) learning resource centers, and (8) college newspapers and publication departments.

In order to gain the support of individuals in the previous areas, speech-language pathologists should expect to attend meetings, strive for social interaction, and act in a manner that will inspire confidence and trust. Although speech-language pathologists may feel their clinical services are of paramount importance, wisdom demands that they give consideration to the needs and objectives of all the college programs. Reasonable requests and expectations insure harmonious relationships with others who also want to attain the goals of their programs. The astute speech-language pathologist keeps the broad goals in mind as relationships with others in the college develop.

Good public relations also may be aided by careful attention to maintaining communication. The conscientious speech-language pathologist is prompt in responding to referrals and informs the referral source when the student has been seen and what the decision has been. (A suggested form is in the Appendix.) When referrals are made to other services or agencies, a call or note stating why the student is being referred keeps lines of communication open.

Use of Communication Aides

Communication aides are used in a variety of speech-language clinical settings. In most cases the on-site speech-language pathologist selects, trains, supervises, and evaluates these paraprofessionals. Communication aides in community colleges have duties similar to aides who work in other programs, that is, supplementing the services of the speech-language pathologist. Frequently students act as communication aides at the college level. A special advantage for using students is that usually they are peers of those they are tutoring. As peers they can help develop socialization skills for those students who need to learn how to make friends and respond in a socially appropriate manner.

Some students elect assignments as communication aides through campus work study programs and receive an hourly wage. Many communication aides are student volunteers who express an interest in the field of speech-language pathology. Others receive credit for field practice in speech-language pathology classes.

Some community colleges have two-year certification programs for training special education aides. Training programs for certification of communication aides are being developed in some community colleges, e.g. Communication Aide: Handicapped Services Option, Pasadena City College. Students take courses in speech-language-hearing disorders, voice and diction, psychology, and special education. Part of the training is working with communicatively handicapped students under the supervision of a qualified speech-language pathologist. Some students in this program become communication aides, while others transfer into university speech-language programs. These students bring with them to the university programs a sophistication as a result of this background experience.

BASES OF A VIABLE SPEECH-LANGUAGE PROGRAM

Administrative Support

The interest in speech-language programs in community colleges is growing, and it is predicted there will be an increase in services for the handicapped as governmental agencies emphasize the equal opportunity trend and provide funds for implementing services to the handicapped. This program is still in its infancy; its potential is just now being evaluated.

When establishing a new program or attempting to expand an existing one, it is necessary to have administrative support. It must be remembered that most administrators do not have the same orientation as those in the speech-language profession; therefore, they must be educated to the needs and benefits of the program. The information administrators use in making program assistance decisions is discussed in Chapter 8. Although the focus of that discussion is university training programs, many of the points covered are applicable to community college settings and others may be modified.

In community colleges, speech-language services are affiliated with various departments and programs: (1) speech, (2) handicapped services, (3) language arts, (4) special services, (5) student personnel, (6) physically handicapped, (7) literature and language, and (8) special education. As an adjunct area to an unrelated program or department, speech and language services may encounter problems with maintaining an appropriate identity. A suggested organizational structure is presented in Figure 5.

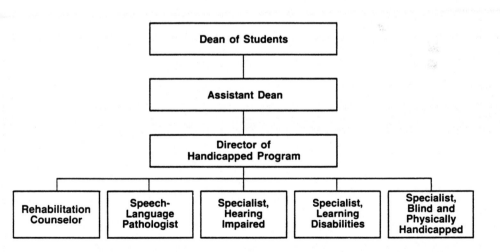

Figure 5. Organizational model for special services. From L. Breakey, S. Kesterson, B. Price, and L. Rasmussen, Community Colleges and the Speech Pathologist. California Speech and Hearing Association Annual Convention, March 27, 1977, San Francisco, California.

The location of speech-language services within the structure of the college is important. In the model presented, the director focuses attention on special services for the handicapped. As dean of student services, this director has background in both academic and clinical services. His responsibility is to all special service coordinators, thus unifying the services offered by each specialist.

Community support for the program is desirable. An advisory committee of respected professionals, leading business executives, and prominent local politicians can be persuasive in helping administrators evaluate realistically the benefits of the program. Community involvement frequently offers tangible benefits. Many service organizations are committed to helping the handicapped. They may give not only moral support to projects but also financial assistance. Some organizations have donated vans for the physically handicapped, video caption boxes for the deaf, and Language Masters® and specialized program materials for the speech-language handicapped.

Facilities

Physical plants vary from one site to another. In some colleges the available facilities are impressive, and in others they are minimal. Facilities used for speech-language services should be suited to the needs of students and staff with emphasis on students receiving effective professional services under conditions commensurate with efficiency, safety, comfort, and privacy. Important considerations include the following:

1. Facility of adequate size, which permits privacy and is relatively free from extraneous noise
2. Facility properly heated or cooled with adequate lighting and ventilation
3. Facility furnished for the type of services offered
4. Locked cabinets and adequate storage space for materials, equipment, and books
5. Rooms readily accessible to nonambulatory students

Suggestion: If appropriate space is not available, a mobile unit may be the solution.

Minimum standards have been established by the American

Speech-Language-Hearing Association (ASHA, 1969).

Some colleges have facilities beyond the minimum requirements, and the most impressive suites contain therapy rooms, audiological soundproof rooms, group therapy rooms, waiting area, offices for speech-language pathologists, secretarial space, and storage area for equipment, materials, and books. This allows for the greatest flexibility in scheduling and serving students.

Campus and Community Resources

Campus Services

An effective speech-language program requires careful attention to ways of using the services offered on a community college campus. No college ever has enough speech-language pathologists, large enough facilities, or all the equipment and materials necessary for the ideal program; however, every community college has an abundance of related services that may be used to enhance and individualize the speech-language program.

Learning disabilities programs under the direction of learning disability specialists are related and allied services to the speech-language program. In the area of language, the learning disability program and the speech-language program interface; the speech-language pathologist is primarily involved in oral communication skills, and the learning disability specialist is concerned mainly with academic proficiency. Since many students require the services of both programs, it is important that the two specialists coordinate their efforts and share diagnostic information and goals and objectives. Ideally the programs should share adjoining suites, thus allowing students to move from one area to the other for appointments, therapy, tutoring, and so forth.

Learning resource centers are an effective means of providing instructional and remedial services for all students. The availability of special videotapes, recorder cassettes, braille materials, special instructional materials, and tutors have aided many students who otherwise would have failed without this special help. This center can be particularly beneficial for multiply handicapped students who need special aids for learning. Foreign students can benefit from lessons that provide a structured model. The advantage of the learning resource center is that it enables students to schedule individualized periods of instruction at their convenience.

Health services should be utilized by the speech-language pathologist when appropriate. On some campuses students are referred to the nurse for hearing screening. The nursing staff is a source for medical information and medical resources available within the community.

Tutorial centers can be used to recruit communication aides for the speech-language program. Tutors also can help students who have difficulty in certain courses by assisting them to achieve academic success at the same time they are improving their communication skills.

Counseling centers provide an important service that may supplement the work of the speech-language pathologist. Academic or social problems may interfere with the speech-language progress of some students. Both professional and peer counseling may be recommended for students in need of such additional assistance.

Physical education departments have many excellent courses that provide helpful activities for handicapped students. Students have become active both socially and physically through jogging, swimming, and dancing programs. There are an increasing number of adaptive physical education classes offered for the physically handicapped, which have been helpful in teaching them to maximize their body usage.

Handicapped services offer necessary assistance to aid individual students with specific needs. Using these services helps the speech-language pathologist implement a rounded program. The extent of such services will vary from campus to campus, but generally the following are available: interpreters, orientation programs, loader services (blind), mobility assistance, orthopedic equipment repair, parking permits, housing assistance, and transportation on and off campus.

Career centers are another source for enriching the speech-language program. All campuses have a vocational counseling center, and students can be encouraged to seek professional assistance to learn where their strengths, interests, and talents lie in terms of occupational pursuits. Students who have a sense of direction in pursuing an occupation or profession are goal oriented in improving their communication skills.

Student centers sponsor orientation meetings for new students. At these meetings the services of the speech-language pathologist can be announced and students asked to fill out questionnaires indicating their interest in scheduling an interview with the speech-language pathologist.

Clubs and organizations on campus may be interested in promoting the services of the speech-language program. Some student service clubs seek a project to sponsor, and members may volunteer assistance by acting as receptionists and answering the telephone in the speech-language clinic. Clubs and organizations can provide social interaction for students in the speech-language program.

Psychological services are provided for individuals in the academic environment. The speech-language pathologist may find students whose emotional problems are so pervasive that they impede progress in remediating communication disorders. Referring the student to the psychologist may be indicated.

The speech-language pathologist should investigate all resources on campus and utilize them to enrich the services provided students in the program.

Community Services

Knowledge of services and agencies available within the community is essential for the speech-language pathologist who wishes to develop an effective program at the community college level. The following is a sampling of agencies and services that may be utilized within the community.

Hospital departments of rehabilitation offer speech-language therapy, audiological testing, occupational therapy, physical therapy, and rehabilitative counseling. This setting may be a referral source for students who need more extensive treatment than is available on campus or for those who are unable to participate in regularly scheduled campus programs.

State departments of rehabilitation have resources at their command to provide specialized diagnostic services, therapeutic services, counseling, and financial assistance. Knowledge of the function of the department enables the speech-language pathologist to help students obtain necessary services.

The Social Security Administration is a valuable funding source for handicapped students. On occasion, the speech-language pathologist will encounter a student whose disabilities are such that the individual is unemployable and eligible for disability compensation, which is funded by this federal agency. Knowing the procedure for applying to the Social Security Administration is helpful when counseling a handicapped student.

Local high schools are a readily available source of information on students' academic background. To plan appropriate remediation techniques, the speech-language pathologist will find it beneficial to know the high school personnel and the types of special education programs in which students have been enrolled. When high school personnel are familiar with the services at the post secondary level, they can direct their students to programs and services available at the community college.

Mental health agencies serve individuals in need of specialized counseling and psychological treatment. To expedite referrals, it is helpful if the speech-language pathologist knows the mental health agencies within the community.

National and State Organizations for the Handicapped schedule annual conventions and regional and local conferences. Participation in these conferences enables both speech-language pathologists and handicapped students to obtain current information on the status of handicapped individuals in education and society. This also is an opportunity for the speech-language pathologist to interact and exchange information with specialists from other campuses.

The community services discussed here are not meant to include all available services. The conscientious speech-language pathologist will become knowledgeable of other community resources that students may use to further their professional and personal objectives.

CONCLUSION

The community college setting offers an opportunity and challenge for speech-language pathologists now in the profession and for those entering the profession in the next few years. Rather than coming into an area that has fixed guidelines and procedures to follow, it is an opportunity to pioneer and develop programs and guidelines. As community colleges increase services for handicapped students, more speech-language pathologists will be needed on campus to provide clinical services for a larger number of students who are in both day and evening classes. With an expanded awareness of communication handicapping conditions, there will be an increased interest in courses in voice and diction, lipreading, introduction to speech-language pathology, and others. Aggressive speech-language pathologists should find the community college a stimulating and rewarding setting.

PART III
THE UNIVERSITY

OVERVIEW:
SIDE THREE OF THE TRIAD

Part III is addressed to the final side of the TRIAD. The role of the university faculty in effecting a meaningful experience for all members of the TRIAD is delineated.

Chapter 8 discusses university support, faculty commitment, and faculty responsibilities. Student teaching policies, such as establishing student prerequisites and recruiting faculty with experience in public schools, are outlined in this chapter.

Chapter 9 is divided into two points of focus: (1) duties and responsibilities for administrating an effective student teaching program and (2) the role of supervisory faculty who oversee the student teaching experience. Practical suggestions are given for implementation of student teaching policies and implementation of supervision responsibilities.

The first part of Chapter 9 gives information on screening student teaching applicants, selecting school districts, and developing a working relationship with supervisory personnel. It also describes in detail the administrative duties specific to each member of the TRIAD—student clinician, master clinician, and supervisor. The second part of the chapter defines the role and discusses duties of the supervisor who maintains ongoing dialogue between university and school. This section contains practical information covering a broad spectrum from the role of the supervisor in observations, conferring with student clinicians and master clinicians, to maintaining an effective relationship with school personnel.

Chapter 10 is unique in that it contains information describing course content for a class offered concurrently with student teaching, *Proseminar: Speech-Language-Hearing in the Schools*. It includes suggestions for lecture and discussion topics, student activities, student self-assessment, and special events. The discussion in this chapter focuses on a course whose basic purpose is guiding student clinicians through the student teaching experience.

Chapter 8

UNIVERSITY POLICIES
AND RESPONSIBILITIES

Colleges and universities throughout the country have the formidable assignment of training speech-language pathologists
who are qualified and competent to evaluate and remediate speech,
language, and hearing handicapped children and adults. The university is obligated to train students to become knowledgeable,
skilled representatives of its training program and to be a credit to
the profession. The reputation of a training institution is dependent upon the level of competence attained by the students who
complete the program; therefore, it is incumbent upon universities to offer comprehensive and high calibre programs.

When a college or university approves a program in speech-
language pathology, it is the responsibility of that institution to
support all facets of the program for which approval has been
given, e.g. B.A./B.S., M.A./M.S., Ph.D., ASHA CCC, state licensing, and state certification for the schools.

Training institutions that have been approved by state boards of
education to prepare students for certification in the schools have
three basic components in their program: (1) academic course
work, (2) clinical practicum on campus, and (3) student teaching.
This, too, is a TRIAD in which the three parts are necessary for the
professional training of students for a specific work environment.

It is the responsibility of the speech-language pathology faculty
to develop and implement an academic and clinical program that
meets the requirements for state certification. State boards of
education or some other designated state agency establishes minimum training requirements for speech-language pathologists in
the schools. These mandated requirements should not be considered the ultimate goal of a training program but should be used as
guidelines that represent the base on which a program of the
highest calibre is built.

University administrators have the responsibility to know, understand, and support all components in the approved program. Support comes through three avenues: maintaining morale; providing adequate funding for space, supplies, equipment, and clerical assistance; and allocation of sufficient faculty positions to implement the curriculum and practicum at a professional level of preparation.

FACULTY COMMITMENT

Support and interest of the entire faculty is necessary if students are to be trained adequately for the school assignment. Students who elect the educational setting have chosen a challenging site for employment. In many instances school speech-language pathologists are speech and language specialists for one or more sites; therefore, their training must be comprehensive and prepare them to function competently in what may be considered an isolated environment. They do not have others in their profession nearby to turn to in time of need. They must be self-sufficient, capable of working with the total range of speech-language-hearing disorders, and interact effectively with many different personalities.

The one major requirement that sets the school certification program apart from the other options within the training program is student teaching. The speech-language pathology faculty as a whole must believe in the importance of the student teaching experience if the *intent* of the state mandate is to be fulfilled. In some academic settings student teaching is relegated to a position of secondary status, whereas it should be viewed as an essential component of the total training program. Student teaching is the culmination of the course work and clinical experiences students have completed in the program. In many cases, it is their first opportunity to have practicum experience in an actual work setting outside the sheltered environment of the campus. The importance of academic course work is not under scrutiny, it serves as the theoretical base for all speech-language pathologists; however, the ability to implement effectively this knowledge in a work environment is the ultimate goal of training programs. Too often, supervision of students in the schools is viewed as making a lesser contribution to the program as a whole than teaching the academics. Ideally there should not be a hierarchy placed on activities within the training program; each fulfills a specific purpose.

UNIVERSITY SUPPORT

Education of Administrators

Implementation of a credible speech-language pathology program is dependent upon university administrative support. The first step in gaining such support is to educate administrators to the objectives and purposes of the program. University administrators have no difficulty in understanding the relevance of a lecture course, a seminar, and a science laboratory: but clinical practicum may be out of the area of their experience and out of the realm of their comprehension. It is necessary, therefore, for administrators to understand the relevance and importance of the total practicum unit of the program.

The speech-language pathology faculty, particularly the director of the program, should be knowledgeable of the factors that influence administrators to make decisions favorable to the speech-language program. They also should be cognizant of the constraints under which administrators must work. An informed administrator is more likely to be a receptive administrator. When faculty approach an administrator who has limited knowledge of the program, much valuable time is spent in laying the groundwork, but time spent in the education of administrators may pay dividends at a later date. Suggested methods and information to educate administrators include the following:

1. Informational discussions
   a. General progress of the program on campus
   b. Objectives and criteria established by state and federal agencies
   c. Future directions of the profession
2. Visitations to the speech-language-hearing clinic
   a. Observing clients with speech and language disorders receiving therapy (this is more informative than describing the various types of cases)
   b. Seeing facilities and equipment

3. Periodic reports can be beneficial in a number of ways:
    a. Requires faculty to review the program objectively
    b. Puts data on record to be retrieved when needed
    c. Provides faculty with a better sense of direction: where they have been and where they hope to go
    d. Forces faculty to take a hard look at the strengths and weaknesses of the program
    e. Allows faculty to research programs in other institutions

Not to be overlooked is educating colleagues from other departments. In institutions with strong faculty governance, requests for program changes and financial support are sent to various faculty committees. Colleagues who have understanding and respect for the speech-language pathology program may be on influential committees and can support the request of the program.

Budget and Funding

A university is allotted a prescribed budget to operate all approved academic programs and projects. Administrators must make decisions regarding the allocation of these funds to the many departments on campus. As a result, some speech-language pathology programs receive sufficient funding to implement the objectives of the program, whereas programs on other campuses receive minimal financial backing. When a faculty agrees that its allotted budget should be increased, they are, in essence, requesting administrators to give the speech-language pathology program a higher priority.

What information do administrators consider persuasive in making a favorable decision? Administrators at various levels of the academic community, department chairs, school deans, university deans, vice-presidents, and presidents, have commented on the factors that are most persuasive in winning additional budgetary support for a program. Following is a summation of the information they consider important in making decisions:

1. Increased student enrollment is strong justification for additional budgetary support. When the program has been operating at a fixed budget for a period of time, it is diffi-

cult to justify additional financing unless there is increased enrollment.

2. Studies of the job market may support requests for additional funding. If manpower studies support a need for speech-language pathologists, administrative responses will be more favorable than if such studies show the market is flooded. If a need for these professionals in the community or nation exists and is predicted, it is expected that student enrollment will increase.

3. Does the training of students lead to a productive professional career? In other words, what will graduates from the program be doing in the future?

4. Many administrators look for well-balanced programs. Most administrators favor speech-language programs in which there is a balance between traditional theoretical academics and practicum, which results in competent clinical professionals being trained.

5. A comparison of what is being offered in programs on other campuses is viable information to present.

6. Accreditation requirements of state, regional, and national organizations carry an impact.

7. Input from former students regarding the quality of the program can be an important factor.

8. Input from employers regarding performance of former students can be of value.

9. Welfare of the clients in the campus Speech-Language-Hearing Clinic is a factor.

10. New developments in the profession, which mandate curriculum modification, can be persuasive.

11. Innovative options in the program, which will attract students to the institution, will be viewed favorably by administration.

12. The credibility of the director of training with administrators is an influential factor.

13. A strong advisory committee composed of respected professionals, leading business executives, and prominent local politicians is recommended. One of the most valuable and often overlooked sources of support is the community. Pub-

lic relations often accomplishes positive results. When the community supports the objectives of the program, the issue of faculty self-interest is minimized. Administrators are more likely to listen when there is influential outside support.

There is one approach that is likely to lead to a negative decision. Often the first impulse is to speak to the advantages of upgrading the quality of a program because the faculty believes the level of training should be improved. Every discipline has the desire to upgrade its training program; administrators encounter this facet of academia every day. This approach in and of itself is routine, competitive, and usually futile.

It is imperative that the faculty prepare a well-organized, well-documented presentation, which includes objectives to be attained, rational for implementing stated objectives, and supportive evidence.

Budget support should include funds specific to student teaching:

1. Reimbursement for telephone calls
2. Mileage reimbursement, parking fees, and lodging when overnight travel is required
3. Time and travel reimbursement for supervisors to meet with colleagues from other institutions
4. Exchange of personnel between universities and school districts.

The preceding section contains guidelines for gaining support to implement high calibre programs. Each campus is unique in its organizational structure, and innovative faculties will develop additional persuasive justifications for program support.

STUDENT TEACHING POLICIES

In order to maintain academic integrity, the speech-language faculty develops policies to implement the goals and objectives of the program. It follows, therefore, that the entire faculty should be involved in establishing those policies relevant to student teaching. Such policies encompass general categories: (1) recruitment of faculty, (2) requirements for faculty supervisors, students, and master clinicians, and (3) budgetary support.

Recruitment of Faculty

"The success of any program is probably less dependent upon planning and administration than upon the particular individuals participating in the program" (Conference on Standards for Supervised Experience for Speech and Hearing Specialists in Public Schools, 1969, p. 30).

Policies should be established to recruit full-time faculty who have had extensive public school experience. The advantages of using full-time tenured faculty as opposed to part-time personnel are the following:

1. Full-time faculty know the total program as they have been involved in policy making, curriculum development, and curriculum modifications
2. Full-time faculty are motivated to make long-range plans because they have the security of being a permanent member of the university community
3. Full-time faculty will consider carefully the decisions they make because they will be responsible for implementing these decisions for an extended period of time.
4. Full-time faculty will be on campus more often, as the university is their primary work setting.

Thus, the strengths of a student teaching program are dependent upon "faculty experience, stability, continuity and flexibility" (Monnin & Peters, 1977, p. 105).

There are advantages when faculty are given a combined assignment: student teaching supervision, on-campus clinical supervision, and/or academic classes. When experienced faculty have on-campus contact with students through practicum or course work, they will have identified student behaviors, which may become more visible during the school assignment. Having had contact with students on campus, faculty assigned to school supervision will be more alert to strengths and weaknesses of student clinicians and can be more effective supervisors during the assignment.

A full-time faculty member can reinforce the goals of the training institution with the master clinician. The master clinician should not feel totally responsible for the performance of the student clinician during the school practicum experience. Many master clinicians feel keenly the responsibility they assume when they train students in the school practicum, but the experienced university supervisor can assure the master clinician that, although student teaching is an important element in the training of students, it is but one part of the total training program.

It has been stated previously in this chapter that faculty with school experience should be employed to participate in the student teaching assignment. Faculty members with public school background have the advantage of personally experiencing the achievements, excitement, frustrations, and limitations of working in the school environment. School-experienced university supervisors are familiar with school protocol and procedures and feel secure and confident in this setting. They understand the language and terminology of the schools. It is returning to a familiar environment in a different role. Master clinicians are eager to show off their programs, and these university supervisors have a point of references from their own backgrounds to appreciate the changes in programs and emphasis that have occurred over a period of time.

It is not necessary for master clinicians to apologize for their work settings. The supervisor with a background in the schools probably has worked in less than ideal conditions and knows the frustration of conducting therapy with many distractions.

Experienced supervisors are knowledgeable of what can be accomplished in the school setting. They can evaluate the student's performance in this environment and probably are less likely to accept mediocrity because of their respect for the schools as a challenging work setting.

It is the responsibility of the director of training to see that faculty are hired whose background includes the following:

1. M.A. or Ph.D. in speech-language pathology
2. American Speech-Language-Hearing Association Certificate of Clinical Competence in Speech-Language Pathology
3. State license for speech-language pathologists (if the state has licensure)
4. Public school certification and clinical experience with the following:
   a. Pupils having a wide variety of speech-language-hearing disorders
   b. Pupils from preschool through high school

The director of training appoints a faculty member who meets the preceding criteria to act as coordinator for the student teaching program. The coordinator assumes responsibility for implementation of established policies, since it is neither feasible nor desirable for the entire faculty to be involved directly in implementing student teaching policies.

When selecting faculty for supervision of student teaching, the ability to supervise off-campus practicum effectively should be given careful consideration. To be an effective supervisor, the person must possess certain desirable personal and professional qualities (Oratio, 1977, pp. 90–91). Essential personal and professional characteristics include the ability to be both objective and perceptive. From the *Conference on Standards for Supervised Experience for Speech and Hearing Specialists in Public Schools,* the following qualities were identified as being desirable: flexibility; tolerance for differences of opinion; clinical expertise; respect for the schools as a setting for speech-language-hearing services; understanding and respect for the roles of administrators, teachers, specialists, etc.; a willingness to learn and change opinions of the nature of educational and therapeutic processes; and a high degree of interest in the growth of the student (1969, pp. 31–32).

Supervisors must enjoy meeting people. They must enjoy selling the training program. It is also helpful if they enjoy driving. "Have map, will travel" is the slogan for university supervisors.

Requirements for the TRIAD

Faculty should establish policies for each of the TRIAD members in order to maintain academic integrity, professional standards, and continuity of programming.

Coordinator/Supervisor

Policy should be established that provides a method for the coordinator of student teaching to report regularly with information to the faculty as a whole. Speech-language pathology faculty should be kept informed of developments in school programs so they may make appropriate modifications in curriculum and clinical training.

Policy should emphasize frequent on-site observations by the faculty appointed to supervision. Most supervisors are conscientious, hard working, and self-directed, and they make several visits on site to observe student clinicians. Unfortunately, situations exist in which university supervisors do not supervise (O'Toole, 1973). Some students are sent into a school setting where the university supervisor never appears on site for observations. The student and master clinician are left to manage as best they can. The amazing part of this situation is that districts continue to accept students under these adverse conditions. It attests to the professional commitment of the master clinician but says little for the professional commitment of those university faculty.

Students

The speech-language pathology faculty establishes policy relative to student requirements for participation in the program, including (1) academic and clinical prerequisites for student teaching, (2) acceptable personal and professional qualities, (3) minimum experiences required for satisfactory completion of the assignment, and (4) minimum level of competence to be achieved for credit to be assigned.

Master Clinicians

The speech-language pathology faculty also establishes policy regarding personal and professional qualifications for master clinicians. A detailed discussion of qualifications considered necessary for speech-language pathologists who participate in the training of student clinicians is found in Chapter 6.

To assist master clinicians in carrying out the responsibilities of the student teaching assignment, faculty should develop policy for planning and conducting in-service training. In-service meetings and workshops are discussed in greater detail in Chapter 9, as they are the direct responsibility of the coordinator of student teaching. The entire faculty, however, should be willing to support these activities by offering suggestions, voting funds from department monies, showing interest in the planning, attending the meetings and workshops, and so forth. Most master clinicians are sincere and conscientious in their desire to do the best job possible, but they need the assistance and support of the faculty in carrying out duties assigned them.

Budgetary Support

Adequate funding is necessary to operate an effective program, and speech-language pathology faculty must be willing to establish policy that makes available a percentage of the department budget for student teaching. Funding should be adequate to cover the costs of (1) clerical assistance, (2) supplies, (3) workshops, (4) in-service training, (5) guest lecturers and (6) special events. If the coordinator of student teaching has a specified budget, the operation of the program can be planned in advance to insure reaching the long-term objectives established by the faculty.

RESPONSIBILITIES

Advisement

Speech-language pathology majors are enrolled in a complex program fulfilling university requirements for a degree, ASHA CCC, state licensure, and/or school certification; therefore, thorough advisement is essential. The faculty has the professional responsibility to aid students in moving expeditiously through the program options they have chosen. Former students have attested that time spent with a knowledgeable adviser has made the difference between moving through a program in the prescribed time and finding oneself deficient two units at graduation time.

The complexity of advisement makes it beneficial to designate certain faculty to advise in specific areas. Those designated to advise in the area of school certification have the responsibility to know and understand current state and university certification requirements. Considerable time and attention is required to keep abreast of the newest developments, but this is necessary if students are to receive proper advisement.

Many students who elect state certification do so without knowing or understanding the role and duties of a speech-language pathologist in the schools. The adviser has the opportunity to describe job responsibilities, to discuss employment opportunities, to inform students of academic and clinical requirements for attaining state certification, and to tell them the purpose and obligations of student teaching. Frequently faculty forget how naive or uninformed a beginning student is. Can they remember back to the days when they, too, were naive students?

It is the responsibility of the faculty to apprise students of the general categories on which they will be evaluated for admission to the student teaching program. Although grades are given due consideration, they do not reflect all the qualities necessary for a student teaching assignment, and students should understand this. Students should be informed of the criteria that are used to determine eligibility for admission to student teaching as established by each university program.

Students have many questions regarding the specifics of the student teaching assignment. Faculty should be prepared to inform students of the basic requirements, for example, how many days a week, how many hours a day, and how long a period of time are required in the assignment. With this information, students can (1) organize course work commitments, (2) arrange transportation, (3) make financial arrangements, (4) plan work schedules, and so forth.

Faculty are aware that student advisement is necessary, but there is another factor that is equally important—counseling. Conscientious faculty will incorporate advisement-counseling into their schedule, for example, students should know how their progress in the program is evaluated by the faculty. Good students are constantly striving to improve and surpass minimum standards, and it is a pleasure to share positive information with these students. Poor students frequently do not have the insight to realize their performance is below expectation. Even when counseled, they do not hear what is being said to them; their defenses are high, and they are unable to comprehend that they are performing below minimum standards. It has been observed that students who consistently ask for specific examples of their poor performance are not able to generalize and usually remain problem students both in the academic environment and in the school setting. Faculty must be aware that such students require special counseling.

Screening

Screening students for the student teaching assignment is one of the most difficult tasks the speech-language pathology faculty undertakes, but it is a professional responsibility they must be willing to assume and perform with diligence. The purpose of screening is twofold: (1) to ascertain that all academic and clinical prerequisites have been met and (2) to assess past performance as a predictor of success in the school assignment. In the screening process, student applications are approved, postponed, or denied. When faculty approve of the candidates, that indicates they are representative of the calibre of student the university considers a credit to the program. Implementation of screening procedures is described in Chapter 9.

The faculty should not look to off-campus personnel to do their screening for them. When a student is given an off-campus assignment, the university gives its seal of approval and says to off-campus personnel, "This student represents our program." The university is implying to the off-campus speech-language pathologist that, based on campus performance, the student has the potential to succeed in the school assignment. There are some students who will have performed competently in classes and in the campus speech-language clinic and who appear ready for the school setting. Not all will be successful in the student teaching assignment. Misjudgments in screening will occur, but most off-campus personnel are understanding of such situations when they realize the faculty tries to avoid such occurrences.

Supporting the TRIAD

The involvement of the speech-language pathology faculty in the student teaching program is evident in several tangible ways: developing curriculum, establishing policies, and selecting qualified personnel. There is one more area where faculty commitment is needed, and that is the intangible area of moral support for personnel directly involved in the student teaching assignment.

For the student teaching program to be effective, it is imperative that the faculty, both individually and collectively, support established policies. Students have been known to shop around until they hear answers they find compatible with their personal interests. The authority of faculty responsible for implementing policy is only as effective as the unified support of the faculty. It is frustrating to hear a student say, "Professor Jellyfish said it was O.K. with him if it is all right with you if I . . ." Such situations undermine the authority of other faculty members. This gives Professor Jellyfish the halo effect while you look like the demon with horns. Or, Professor Lockjaw, who voted in the minority against a particular policy, now refuses to support it based on principle. It does not take students long to realize there may be something to be gained by playing one professor against another. Valuable time, effort, and energy must be spent in resolving issues that never should have surfaced in the first place. With total faculty support, there is consistency in enforcing policies and procedures. This gives students a sense of confidence in their contacts with faculty and unified effort allows the faculty to address themselves to the maintenance and improvement of the quality of education to which they are committed.

Support for Supervisors

When the program is going well, an expression of approval by the faculty to the supervisors is appreciated. When problem areas develop, supervisors gain an inner strength when they know the faculty supports their efforts no matter how stressful the current situation may be.

It is important for the faculty to be *united* in support of the supervisor; a willingness to corroborate and to defend actions taken in implementing student teaching policy is essential. *Esprit de corps* gives strength to the student teaching program.

Support for Master Clinicians

It is expected that the university faculty will show confidence in the master clinicians' abilities to guide, train, and evaluate the performance of students assigned to them. If a master clinician is considered sufficiently competent to assume responsibility as a team member in the training of a student, then as a professional that person deserves the support of the faculty. The master clinician's endorsement of the performance of a student clinician states that the student is meeting the professional level of competence established by the master clinician. Conversely, when a master clinician expresses professional concerns about a student, it is incumbent upon the faculty to respect the concerns voiced by the master clinician. Unfortunately, there have been instances when the concerns of master clinicians have gone unheeded. They are credible speech-language pathologists, whose observations should be given professional consideration.

Support for Students

The speech-language pathology faculty is interested in their students, has an investment in their success, and is supportive of their endeavors to gain professional competence. The faculty should show respect for the students' right to request consideration of individual concerns. There may be situations in which the particular school assignment is not in the student's best interest. They should be able to express their concerns and know they will be given a fair hearing and full consideration by the faculty.

Sometimes there may be circumstances that warrant special consideration. Requests for departure from the rules must be reviewed in terms of the individual, for example, the student's needs and ability to reach the desired level of competence. The request also must be evaluated as setting a precedent that may not be desirable for the good of the overall program. Policies and procedures are established because they are appropriate at the time they are adopted; however, they should be reviewed routinely, and relevant modifications should be made periodically.

CONCLUSION

The strength of the student teaching program is dependent upon the commitment of the total speech-language pathology faculty to the school practicum. Faculty demonstrate their involvement by giving tangible and intangible support to their liaison member, the coordinator of student teaching; establishing policy pertinent to the assignment; helping to educate administrators; voting funding; and supporting the efforts of supervisors, master clinicians, and student clinicians. Strong faculty support for the program promotes cooperation and respect between the training institution and the school setting, thus giving direction to all who participate in the TRIAD.

Chapter 9

COORDINATOR/SUPERVISOR
OF SCHOOL PRACTICUM

There are many ways to implement the student teaching policies established by the speech-language pathology faculty. This chapter will present some suggested procedures to aid coordinators and supervisors in the implementation process.

COORDINATOR

As discussed in Chapter 8, it is not practical for all faculty to be involved in the administrative duties of the student teaching program; therefore, one member is delegated by the director of training to coordinate and implement the various phases of the program. No matter how well student teaching policy is written, a successful program is dependent upon the effectiveness of the coordinator.

The coordinator's duties in the student teaching program will vary according to the size of the program; in small programs the coordinator acts as both coordinator and supervisor, while in large programs the coordinator may act in an administrative capacity only, leaving the actual supervision of student teaching to a team of faculty members.

To implement the student teaching program effectively, the coordinator must be involved with administrative duties. This encompasses responsibilities to the university training program, supervisors, master clinicians, and student clinicians. All administrative assignments require endless hours of paperwork, and this appointment is no exception. Preparing for the actual student teaching assignments begins long before students arrive on site and continues beyond the last day. Included in this area are the following:

1. Screening
   a. Processes applications
   b. Requests faculty input
   c. Presents information to faculty
   d. Acts on faculty decisions
2. Assignments
   a. Contacts districts
   b. Selects master clinicians
   c. Assigns students to master clinicians
   d. Assigns students to university supervisors
3. Duties specific to students
   a. Conducts orientation for prospective student clinicians
   b. Notifies students of placements
   c. Documents clinical hours
   d. Places evaluations on file
4. Duties specific to master clinicians
   a. Notifies master clinicians of students' names, addresses, and telephone numbers
   b. Disseminates information regarding university requirements and other information pertinent to the assignment
   c. Sends guidelines, evaluation forms, and student autobiographies
   d. Oversees the sending and returning of evaluations
   e. Notifies master clinicians of name and telephone number of university supervisor
5. Duties specific to supervisors
   a. Orients new supervisors to the assignment
   b. Sends copies of students' autobiographies to supervisor
   c. Disseminates master clinicians' names, addresses, and telephone numbers to supervisors
   d. Distributes to supervisors students' schedules and directions to schools
   e. Meets periodically with supervisors
6. In-service meetings and workshops
   a. Plans programs
   b. Schedules activities
   c. Distributes announcements
   d. Arranges for publicity
   e. Host the program

Screening

Information on the applicants for student teaching must be compiled thoroughly if appropriate faculty decisions are to be made. The screening process is a three phase operation: (1) preliminary review of applicants, (2) input from faculty, and (3) review and final decisions.

Phase One

The coordinator oversees the review of applicants to confirm that basic requirements have been met: prerequisite courses, clinical hours, grade point average, medical clearance, and so forth.

Phase Two

The coordinator requests input from regular and part-time faculty to aid in assessing each candidate's potential for success in the student teaching experience. Three or more weeks before the faculty is scheduled to review candidates, the coordinator distributes an assessment sheet containing the names of all applicants. It has been found helpful to rate each applicant on a three-point scale: (1) serious concerns, (2) some concerns, and (3) no concerns.

Students who receive all 3s require no further follow-up. When a student receives one or more 2s, the coordinator contacts the faculty who assigned the rating to learn the nature of the concerns, which are then brought to the attention of the entire faculty. If a student receives one or more 1s, the coordinator is alerted that a thorough discussion of the student's performance in the program is necessary. All available information should be compiled to aid the faculty in making an equitable decision.

Phase Three

Final decisions are the responsibility of the regular full-time faculty based on the information collected and submitted by the coordinator.

The majority of applicants receive unqualified approval by faculty. Some applicants will receive approval with reservation. When this occurs, it is desirable for an adviser to have a discussion with the student. When there are significant concerns, it may be appropriate for two or three of the faculty to confer with the student, thus enabling the student to receive input from more than one person. Often a frank discussion before the assignment commences allows the student an opportunity to overcome undesirable behaviors and alerts the student to deficiencies that if not corrected, may become problems during the assignment.

When there are serious concerns of sufficient magnitude to deny a student admittance to student teaching, it is recommended that a subcommittee of the faculty meet with the student. At this meeting the student is informed of the reasons for denying admission to student teaching, options available to the student, and the competencies to be achieved before reapplying for student teaching. Meeting with a subcommittee is less intimidating for the student than meeting with the faculty as a whole, and frequently, a more productive discussion takes place. In some instances, however, meeting with the entire faculty may be advisable. Following such a conference, it is recommended that a letter be sent to the student summarizing the main points discussed. During the conference, the student's anxiety level may have been so great or defenses so high that much of what had been said was not absorbed. Having a copy of the letter on file provides a record of the problems that existed and the conditions set forth. This is protection for both the student and the faculty if a decision regarding student teaching is to be made at a later time.

Assignments

The coordinator is responsible for making the student teaching assignments. This encompasses a broad spectrum of duties—selecting school districts and master clinicians, contacting district administrators, and assigning students to master clinicians and university supervisors. Some university programs assign all their students to one or two districts, and placement procedures, therefore, are consistent and greatly simplified. Other training programs utilize the services of many districts; thus, placement procedures must be flexible to conform to the policies of each district. The number of districts used is dependent upon the size of the training program, the availability of qualified master clinicians, and geographic considerations of students and supervisors. By the time students reach this level in their academic programs, they usually are willing to travel to insure themselves an optimum experience, but in fairness to them, distance and weather conditions must be taken into consideration when assignments are made.

As discussed in Chapter 6, speech-language pathologists who possess the professional and personal qualities considered necessary for participation in the TRIAD are selected to become master clinicians. The procedure for the selection of master clinicians depends upon university and district policies. One or more of the following may be utilized: (1) the coordinator may contact the appropriate school administrator requesting placement of students for assignments in the district; the selection of the speech-language pathologist is left to the professional judgment of the administrator, (2) the coordinator may contact the district administrator and request a particular speech-language pathologist to be a master clinician, or (3) the coordinator may contact a speech-language pathologist directly to fulfill this role.

When large school districts are used for placement, some university coordinators meet with school speech and language personnel, and together they select master clinicians, thus establishing a cooperative relationship. If difficulties arise, it is less threatening for either party to pick up a telephone and, on a first-name basis, discuss the problem.

Regardless of how the selection is made, the coordinator involves district administrators in the process of selecting master clinicians. The hallmark of a successful coordinator is the ability to show respect and understanding of procedures and limitations placed upon school personnel, and to show appreciation for their participation in the training program. Before completing arrangements to place a student, contract arrangements are finalized through channels established by the university and districts, which insures the student clinician the legal sanction to be on site as a trainee.

When the coordinator knows the personalities, interests, and professional background of both students and master clinicians, it is possible to bring together those participants who can work cooperatively. Although it is not a prime requirement that master clinicians and students become lifelong friends, establishing an atmosphere of mutual regard and professional understanding enhances the assignment for both parties.

In large university programs when more than one faculty member is responsible for supervision, the coordinator, in consultation with the supervisors, assigns student clinicians to them. An effective coordinator is considerate of the supervisory faculty and takes into account on-campus commitments, geographical locations, and other circumstances before assignments are finalized.

It may be advantageous to have two supervisors assigned to a borderline candidate, as more attention can be given to the student's performance. If the student encounters difficulties, it may be beneficial to have more than one opinion. A team of experts observing the same behaviors makes counseling sessions more productive and negates individual biases and personality conflicts.

The conscientious coordinator meets periodically with school district speech and language personnel to discuss goals and directions regarding the student teaching program. Such an exchange of views is constructive for both university and school personnel.

Duties Specific to Students

The coordinator of student teaching has responsibilities to students prior to, during, and after completion of the assignment. One responsibility is to make certain that candidates are knowledgeable and understand what is expected of them during the school assignment. If students have not received information specific to student teaching in a prerequisite course, an orientation meeting for candidates is recommended. Information should be presented, which includes the following:

1. Guidelines of experiences required for successful completion of the assignment (see Appendix for suggested guidelines)
2. Description of the specific requirements of the assignment
3. Guidelines of personal and professional responsibilities for student clinicians (see Appendix for suggested guidelines)
4. Evaluation forms
5. Recommended readings

Frequently students do not realize the rigorous demands of the assignment. A former student or master clinician describing the expectations has a greater impact on the students than a faculty member who is saying the same thing. The coordinator may wish to invite a master clinician or a former student to describe the responsibilities of the assignment.

Students may have concerns about student teaching that are especially significant to them. The coordinator may be in a position to allay anxieties, to answer questions, or to suggest options. Problems or concerns that can be resolved prior to student teaching will enable the student clinician to perform more effectively once the assignment has begun.

When assignments have been finalized, the coordinator notifies students of the following: (1) the district in which they will do their practicum, (2) the master clinician to whom they are assigned, and (3) the starting and ending dates of the assignment. It is not unusual for the coordinator to let students contact the master clinicians to arrange with them the specifics of the assignment, for example, days of the week. This approach is beneficial because master clinicians know their own case load and the days student clinicians will have the best experiences. When a student is assigned to two school sites with two master clinicians, the master clinicians are in a better position than the university coordinator to arrange the schedule for the student.

At the end of the assignment, master clinicians and university supervisors write a final evaluation for each of the assigned student clinicians. When the evaluation forms are returned by the master clinicians, it is the responsibility of the coordinator to see that these evaluations are made available to the supervisors for counseling with students. If students are scheduled for employment interviews prior to the completion of student teaching, midterm evaluations may be sent to educational placement; otherwise, the coordinator sees that the final evaluations are on file.

Duties Specific to Master Clinicians

The coordinator apprises master clinicians of their duties and responsibilities to student clinicians. This may be accomplished by providing master clinicians with a packet of information prior to the student's arriving for the assignment. Included in the packet are the following:

1. Cover letter thanking master clinician for participation
2. Description of specific requirements of the assignment
3. Master clinician's guidelines
4. Description of university student teaching program
5. Evaluation form
6. Name, address, and telephone number of student clinician
7. Student's autobiography

Familiarity with the material in the packet, particularly with the university student teaching program and the master clinician's guidelines, enables the master clinician to plan in advance how the student will meet the requirements of the assignment.

Master clinicians have attested to the value of having an autobiography from the student prior to the first day. Student's autobiographies should include academic and clinical experiences and ultimate professional goals and objectives. This information gives master clinicians a sense of direction for planning the best experiences for the students.

If master clinicians have a copy of the evaluation form prior to the assignment, they will know in advance the parameters on which the student is to be evaluated. Most university programs require master clinicians to evaluate the student's performance at least twice during the assignment, at midterm and at the end of the semester. It is the coordinator's responsibility to see that these evaluation forms are sent to master clinicians at appropriate times and returned so the evaluations may be placed on file.

The coordinator should be available to assist master clinicians in fulfilling their role in the training of student clinicians. The coordinator should be ready to answer questions and resolve concerns expressed by master clinicians. This may be effected through personal communication, through the university supervisor, or as part of in-service training meetings.

Duties Specific to Supervisors

An important responsibility of the coordinator is to see that new supervisors are oriented into the procedures and expectations of the assignment. The coordinator should help the supervisors put their role in perspective relative to the total training program.

Previous public school background does not predict competence as university supervisors; therefore, they may need help in improving supervisory skills necessary for this assignment. This may be accomplished through discussion and conferences between the coordinator and the supervisory faculty.

Supervisors should be supplied with pertinent information, such as student's schedules, addresses, telephone numbers of schools, directions to schools, names and telephone numbers of master clinicians and students. It is helpful to have this information typed on a five-by-eight card for easy reference. Supervisors also should be given copies of students' autobiographies.

It is not unusual for new supervisors to feel they are totally responsible for the success or failure of a student clinician. Their individual contribution is important, but an understanding coordinator can help them realize they are one of many who influence the student's level of competence. The perceptive coordinator is a good listener but does not hesitate to let supervisors know when they are doing a good job.

In-service Meetings and Workshops

Classroom teachers have expressed their disappointment and lack of respect for in-service meetings (Polite, 1980). The prevailing comments of classroom teachers can be generalized to master clinicians. The astute coordinator will try to avoid making the mistakes discussed by Polite, which contribute to negative comments and resistance to participation. Incorporating the following suggestions when planning in-service programs will aid in generating a receptive attitude: (1) involve supervisors and master clinicians in the planning of in-service programs in order to assure their active participation, (2) choose dynamic participants for program planning and presentation, (3) emphasize the practical features of the programs, (4) insure that in-service training meets the needs of participants and is applicable to their school populations and work settings, and (5) make the evaluation of in-service effectiveness sufficiently detailed so that the participants feel their opinions are given appropriate consideration and will influence planning of future in-service meetings.

The coordinator who schedules in-service meetings and workshops for the members of the school practicum is keeping lines of communication open, which ultimately strengthens the entire student teaching program, as well as providing a method for giving information to all participants in the TRIAD.

The purpose of in-service meetings is to provide a forum for master clinicians and university personnel, which gives the participants an opportunity to (1) define the goals of the total training program, (2) describe how the program is designed to enable students to achieve these goals, (3) delineate the role of the master clinician within the training program, and (4) enable the university to receive feedback on the training program.

Most master clinicians assign a high level of professional significance to their role in training student clinicians (*Conference on Standards for Supervised Experience for Speech and Hearing Specialists in Public Schools,* 1969). Master clinicians often express interest in knowing how their performance is viewed by others; they, too, look for feedback from students and university personnel to aid them in refining their skills. Conducting in-service meetings for master clinicians and university personnel develops a corps of knowledgeable and competent master clinicians for the training program.

The perceptive coordinator is aware of the importance of peer support. In-service meetings provide opportunities for peer interaction among master clinicians, which encourages them to express their individual concerns about handling the specifics of the assignment. In the school setting, often they are isolated and feel their problems are unique; therefore, it is reassuring for them to know their peers have encountered similar problems. They look for answers from experienced master clinicians and university faculty on how to manage the day-to-day questions that arise throughout the student teaching assignment. Master clinicians sometimes are more willing to listen to suggestions from each other in a group setting than they are to accept the same suggestions individually from the university supervisor or coordinator.

Some issues frequently need clarification for master clinicians: (1) how long the student should observe the master clinician, (2) when the student should be given responsibility for the entire case load, (3) who is responsible for the discipline of pupils, (4) how much authority should the student be given, (5) what is the extent to which students should participate in parent and school staff conferences, (6) what is the expected level of competence in assessment and therapeutic procedures of students, and (7) what materials are students expected to develop during the assignment?

Various formats can be used for in-service training: (1) new master clinicians meet for an orientation to discuss their role with the university coordinator, supervisors, and experienced master clinicians, (2) master clinicians meet with the coordinator and supervisors to discuss common concerns, or (3) master clinicians meet with the coordinator, supervisors, and student clinicians to discuss implementation procedures for policies and requirements of the assignment.

All three formats have been employed, and each has been productive in achieving specific objectives. The most successful approach has included all three sides of the TRIAD: university supervisors, master clinicians, and student clinicians. It has been found that small group interaction facilitates a freedom in the flow of communication. If there are a large number of participants, they may be assigned to small groups where topics can be discussed more easily. Each small group is composed of master clinicians, student clinicians, and a university supervisor. It is recommended that the participants be divided so students are not in the same group with their master clinicians. Open discussions take place most readily when personalities and personal commitments are not involved. An agenda of items to be discussed is given to each group so that the discussion focuses upon specific areas of common interest. This format has been most effective when university faculty have assumed the role of observer and resource person. In this situation, it is the intent of university faculty not to influence master clinicians and students in reaching their conclusions but to facilitate interaction. At the end of a designated period, each group reports to the entire gathering the pertinent points exchanged during the small group discussions. The coordinator compiles this information and uses it to strengthen the student teaching program.

Workshops may be scheduled by the coordinator for master clinicians and students, which provide an opportunity to exchange therapeutic approaches and materials. Many speech-language pathologists develop therapeutic procedures that are unique, but frequently they do not appreciate the merit and excellence of their techniques. University supervisors, by virtue of observing many therapy procedures, are in a position to make comparative judgments. University personnel then select outstanding master clinicians to present methods and/or materials at a university-sponsored workshop. In some cases the recognition of their skills has provided some master clinicians with the impetus to pursue publication of their materials and/or to present their techniques at state and national conferences.

Master clinicians who are chosen to make a workshop presentation receive peer and university recognition, which does more for one's ego than a letter of commendation. As a member of the training TRIAD, master clinicians *may* receive an honorarium, which is pitifully small and does not begin to compensate them for the time expended in training students (Willbrand and Tibbits, 1976). Speaking to this point, Vairo and Perel ask, "Can the universities and society expect the cooperating teacher to consider his role important if he is given no recognition, no assistance, and almost no remuneration?" (1973, p. 131). Workshops are a form of recognition by the university and peers for contributions master clinicians make to the training program.

Additional Administrative Duties

One last salute to administrivia! The university coordinator must be a *well-organized* paper pusher! For the student teaching program to be efficient, the coordinator must oversee clerical procedures. Few universities have a secretary whose only assignment is the student teaching program. Sometimes a part-time person is hired to carry out this duty or a graduate student is given this responsibility. This means that office operations must be maintained through the ongoing effort of the coordinator.

A helpful hint is to have a master calendar on which deadlines, dates of events, notices to be sent, and so forth are entered. Whoever is currently in charge of office procedures can anticipate the forms to be mailed, the room reservations to be made, the workshops to be announced, the evaluations to be sent, and so on. It also is helpful to have a master clinician card file containing pertinent information: name, address, telephone number, school district, date, school, and name of student supervised.

The well-organized coordinator makes it possible for all members of the TRIAD to function in an effective manner. It is through the efforts of the coordinator that each TRIAD member can be assured that his role in the student teaching program has the attention from the university that it deserves.

SUPERVISORS

Faculty assigned the supervisory role have a major involvement in the success of the student teaching program. The supervisor is the representative of the university program to the master clinician and other school personnel. Judgments made by school personnel regarding the training program are largely influenced by the impression made by university supervisors. If they are knowledgeable, understanding, concerned, and dependable, there will be a positive reaction to the training program by school personnel. Based on this positive reaction, they will be more willing to provide student clinicians with the best experiences possible and be receptive to accepting students in the future. If the university supervisor displays negative and undesirable personal and professional characteristics, positive relations between school personnel and the training program may be impeded.

Supervisors with school experience have knowledge of how schools operate, which gives them valuable insight into knowing the best ways to communicate with school personnel as well as ways to communicate with student clinicians to bridge the gap between on-campus experience and school practicum.

University supervisors have the responsibility to keep abreast of developments in school speech-language programs. If they know and understand the responsibilities of school speech-language pathologists, they can evaluate better the performance of student clinicians based on the knowledge of both the school and university programs. Supervisors also can assess the adequacy and appropriateness of the training program as preparation for the school experience.

Defining the Role

"Supervision is an involved task but it is basic to good clinical training" (Halfond, 1964, p. 441). Over a period of years many authors have discussed the importance of the supervisory process and the didactic role of the supervisor in clinical practicum (Oratio, 1977; Schubert, 1978; Van Riper; 1965). According to Anderson (1974) special skills are necessary to be a successful supervisor: understanding the clinical process, developing multiple skills in observing behavior, being an expert in communicating feedback, understanding modification of adult behavior, understanding one's strengths and weaknesses as a clinician and as a person, and having the ability to evaluate, encourage, reinforce, coordinate, and moderate. Good university supervisors use these skills in meeting their many responsibilities as a member of the student teaching TRIAD. Some of the responsibilities relevant to student teaching supervision in which these skills should be used are acting as a representative for the university training program, overseeing the experiences student clinicians have in the schools, and sharing information with the coordinator and faculty.

Beyond the general duties stated previously, the main responsibility of the supervisor is overseeing and supervising the clinical performance of the student in the schools. This responsibility requires incorporating the tangible and intangible qualities necessary for good supervision in any setting. Incorporating the supervisor-teacher paradigm makes the difference between being a good supervisor and performing superficially in the role. Supervisors, regardless of the setting, are teachers and should be prepared to instruct. Instructional responsibilities are similar, whether they take place on or off campus. The location of instruction is not as significant as the information that is imparted, for example, holding a conference in a school faculty room is as meaningful as holding a conference in the supervisor's office, and the student has the benefit of immediate feedback.

When faculty accept the supervisory assignment, they should be aware they are assuming responsibilities that are more encompassing than *visiting* the student clinician a few times in the school setting. Student teaching is considered sufficiently important that it is a requirement in every state for school certification, and it requires the same time, effort, and concentration as any other academic and clinical assignment. Students should be given a sense of direction the same as they are in any other learning situation. The same care and attention should be given to the practicum assignment in the schools as is given to developing the student's clinical skills on campus. Supervisors bring to the school practicum assignment the supervisory skills and techniques they have developed and refined in on-campus supervision. Supervisors should use these skills and techniques with students in off-campus practicum settings. Faculty who are engaged in school supervision fulfill their responsibilities to the student clinician, master clinician, and the profession when they become directly involved in contributing to the student's clinical performance.

University supervisors are professionals who are "responsible for the growth, improvement, and development of clinical skills of student clinicians" (Schubert, 1978, p. 3). In the school practicum this responsibility is shared with the master clinician. Although master clinicians are with the students on an ongoing basis, university supervisors have a broad perspective of the total training program goals. Some master clinicians may look to the university supervisor to fulfill a leadership role and to give support to their daily efforts, particularly master clinicians who have had only limited experience with student clinicians. The combination of two competent experienced professionals, each supplementing the contribution of the other, provides the most meaningful experience for the student.

Duties Specific to University Supervisors

Following are some of the duties specific to university supervisors:
1. Observation of student clinicians in the schools
2. Maintenance of a dialogue with student clinicians and master clinicians
3. Evaluation of student clinicians' performance
4. Documentation of supervised hours
5. Public relations with school personnel

Observations

Although "there have been no reports of research on the supervisory process conducted within school based practica" (Caracciola et al., 1980, p. 119), the value of good supervision cannot be overemphasized. Observing in the schools is not merely arriving on site and being a passive recipient of what is happening. Observations by the university supervisor should contribute to a learning situation for students by helping them develop a better sense of direction, gain insight into the role of being a student clinician, and improve skills necessary for becoming a competent speech-language pathologist.

When supervisors arrive at the off-campus setting, they should be prepared to use the supervisory skills developed on campus to the advantage of student clinicians and master clinicians. The most successful off-campus supervision takes place when university faculty are experienced in both on-campus and off-campus practicum supervision. On-campus supervision experience gives supervisors a realistic appraisal of the level of clinical competence beginning clinicians have reached, which enables supervisors to be realistic of the expectations of clinicians beginning the student teaching assignment. Off-campus supervision also makes faculty more effective on-campus supervisors. They are able to see their protégés perform in the school setting. Student strengths observed on campus should be in evidence off campus, and what may have been perceived as minor problems in the campus clinic may be major problems in the field. This experience alerts the supervisor to encourage continued development of strengths and to attempt to correct problem areas before students are sent to off-campus sites. A broad comprehensive frame of reference contributes to better supervision in both environments. At the same time, there is an awareness that in the school practicum, the supervisor has the additional responsibility of interacting with both the student clinician and master clinician.

Frequent visits by the supervisor to the school setting for observations of student clinicians and an exchange of information with master clinicians shows both of them that the school assignment is considered an important part of the training program. How many times should the university supervisor observe on site? There are so many variables in student teaching assignments that it is not possible to state an optimum number. The basic purpose of on-site observations is to evaluate the performance of the student clinician; therefore, visitations should be frequent enough throughout the assignment for the university supervisor to observe growth in the student's performance, to give input to the student, and to evaluate the student's ability to function competently in the school environment. If a student clinician is encountering problems, the university supervisor should schedule additional observations and work closely with the master clinician and student clinician until the problems are resolved.

Some supervisors, master clinicians, and student clinicians prefer unscheduled observations. The advantage of this approach is that the student does not build up anxiety over the planned visit; therefore, sessions observed are more representative of daily performance. The disadvantage is that the supervisor may arrive on a day when there are major changes in the school schedule—field trips, assemblies, and so forth. Most supervisors do not have time for these uncertainties. If visitations are scheduled and there are changes in the school routine, the supervisor can be notified. On scheduled observations, however, the student clinician may have a high level of anxiety and will be trying to impress the supervisor. The astute supervisor will take this into consideration when judging the performance of the student clinician. It is not unusual for the master clinician to experience anxiety. Some of the anxiety will be for the student because master clinicians want their students to perform well. Some of the anxiety will be personal, because the master clinician may believe the student's performance is a reflection of how the master clinician is performing in the assigned role.

As stated earlier, supervisors are most effective when they interact with both master clinicians and student clinicians. The supervisor fulfills this responsibility by conferring with the master clinician and student clinician either individually or together, and time should be allotted for this interaction to take place outside the therapy session. There have been instances in which discussions of students' performances have taken place during the observation. When others in the room are talking, it can be distracting and unnerving for students who know they are the subject of the conversation. This weakens the student clinicians' authority role with the children they are working with and often is damaging to an emerging ego. Considerate supervisors want student clinicians to have every opportunity to demonstrate their competence in the assignment.

Maintaining a Dialogue

Conferences with student clinicians and master clinicians are an integral part of the supervision process. It is through frequent contacts that continuing dialogue is maintained with master clinicians and student clinicians. Conferences will encompass many subjects ranging from questions concerning the logistics of student teaching to in-depth evaluation of the student clinician's overall performance.

University supervisors have opportunities to schedule conference appointments with students both off campus and on campus as the need arises. When the supervisor of the student teaching assignment is also the instructor of the proseminar, this provides additional on-campus opportunities for interaction between the student and supervisor (see Chapter 10).

Conferences may be scheduled to review and clarify with students the requirements of the assignment and to insure they are being met. In some instances the master clinician may not be able to provide all the experiences that the university requires, and it may be necessary to make other arrangements. When reviewing assignment schedules with students, supervisors may become aware of special problems student clinicians are encountering and can help resolve these difficulties early in the student teaching experience.

Supervisors should be prepared to discuss with master clinicians the student teaching program and answer questions relative to all phases of the assignment. Having accepted a student attests to their motivation to fulfill a professional commitment; however, they may be unsure of specific academic expectations. Supervisors are in a position to give them this information and help them define their role as master clinicians.

It is to be expected that first-time master clinicians will have many questions about their responsibilities. Although master clinicians may have been given guidelines and a description of the university requirements, the supervisor should be prepared to discuss and clarify these with master clinicians. Master clinicians may inform supervisors that it is difficult or impossible to provide all the experiences requested by the university. With this information, supervisors can make appropriate modifications of the assignment with the student. Or, the master clinician may suggest experiences that are not part of the requirements but that may enrich the experiences for the student clinician.

Conferences with the master clinician and student clinician usually take place on the school site following the observation. One method of insuring objectivity in the conference is using the student's daily lesson plans as the central focus of the discussion. Both student clinician and master clinician need input from the university supervisor, and both want to share their reactions with the supervisor. Talking together may be advantageous; the three parties involved will know specifically what has been said. Misinterpretations are less likely to occur when a written record of the conference is made, e.g. an anecdotal record or a formal conference report, as indicated.

In some situations it may be advisable to confer with the student clinician and master clinician individually. Individual conferences may produce freer communication, especially if there are problem areas that need to be discussed and resolved. Such conferences may take place on campus, at the school site, or over the telephone. When problems do occur in the assignment, it is helpful to ask the student clinician, or master clinician, as the case may be, to be specific about the concerns. An anecdotal record is a useful means of objectifying the sharing of information. By keeping lines of communication open, the astute supervisor can pinpoint troubled areas and help the student and the master clinician bring the student teaching assignment to a successful conclusion.

In most assignments student clinicians and master clinicians form a positive relationship. There are occasions, however, when personality differences are such that a good working relationship is difficult to maintain. In some cases the supervisor can make suggestions that may help the student and/or the master clinician work through some of the difficult areas. If it is not possible to achieve a working relationship that will enable the student to receive the type and level of experience desired, then the university supervisor must make the decision to assign the student to another setting. Often the thoughtful supervisor can be instrumental in facilitating this decision to be one of mutual agreement with the master clinician and the student clinician. Promptness, tact, and a caring manner help to keep the results of these decisions as positive as possible. Although it is desirable to have assignments that are positive and pleasant for student clinicians, sometimes they can learn by negative experiences. Supervisors can help student clinicians direct their attention to the constructive aspects of what they will not do when they are in a working situation on their own.

Occasionally, the master clinician reports, "Suzi's doing great!" but the supervisor does not agree with this evaluation. What can be done? The tactful supervisor will explore various approaches to resolve the differences in opinion. (1) One approach is to confer with the master clinician and focus the discussion on specific areas of performance. A tactful way to initiate the dialogue is, "I'm glad you see Suzi's strengths. Let's talk about them." "Now, let's discuss areas where Suzi should concentrate on improving." This method is especially helpful if the master clinician has had other student clinicians so a comparison in performance can be made. (2) An evaluation of the student's performance by another university supervisor may be helpful. (3) A third opinion from another experienced master clinician may also be constructive and an objective means of giving the student clinician a fair and realistic evaluation. (4) Invite the district speech-language supervisor to observe and evaluate the student clinician's performance.

Sometimes it may be necessary for the university supervisor to override the evaluation of the master clinician, while in other cases, it may be wisdom to accept the evaluation of the master clinician and walk away knowing that, as a supervisor, you cannot win them all!

Experienced supervisors are aware that master clinicians and student clinicians appreciate positive reinforcement from university personnel. Successful supervisors seek opportunities to find areas for specific commendation. Complimenting participants on their efforts and accomplishments helps insure that dialogue among the TRIAD members is as productive as possible.

Evaluating Student Clinician Performance

Throughout the student teaching assignment, the supervisor is involved in evaluating the performance of the student clinician. Periodic evaluations of student clinicians' performances are based upon their level of competency to fulfill the established criteria of the school experience. The supervisor will obtain information from student clinicians and master clinicians through conversing, reviewing written records, looking at lesson plans, directly observing therapy sessions, and watching the interaction between the student clinician, pupils in the case load, and school personnel.

Some supervisors develop with student clinicians and their master clinicians a set of competencies that student clinicians are to perfect before the assignment is completed. During the observations the supervisor is evaluating the student's level of performance as measured against the established competencies. Supervisors may use one of several approaches for evaluating student competency, for example, asking student clinicians to submit a written self-assessment of their school practicum performance to be turned in prior to the scheduled observation or to assess their performance on the day the supervisor observes. Self-assessment serves as a basis for conferences in which the strengths and weaknesses perceived by the student clinician are compared with the judgments of the supervisor. Or, the supervisor may critique students' performances and ask students to respond to these comments. This may be accomplished in two ways: (1) Conferences are scheduled immediately following the observation in which students respond to the comments and questions raised. The advantage of this method is an immediate exchange of information while the practicum is still fresh in everyone's mind. A disadvantage is that students may not have adequate time to formulate sagacious responses. (2) Conferences are scheduled a week or ten days later, in which students prepare written responses to the comments and questions the supervisor presented during the observation. The latter approach offers learning opportunities for students and gives the supervisor valuable insight into students' abilities to formulate therapy rationale. Competent students will research, investigate, integrate information, and present a theoretical rationale for objectives planned and procedures used, or they will understand the inappropriateness of some of their clinical procedures. Weak students who are unable to develop in-depth rationale will present superficial or inappropriate responses. This insight into students' abilities gives the supervisor a basis for conferring and making value judgments on clinical abilities of student clinicians.

The method of rating students' performances will depend upon the supervisor's preference. Some supervisors assign a letter grade to the observation; others rate it on a scale from 1 to 10; or no grade is given to the observation, and students receive oral and/or written feedback by the university supervisor.

At the end of the assignment, the university supervisor writes a final formal evaluation of each student's clinical performance. This must be a careful and honest appraisal of the student's overall performance in student teaching. Prospective employers look for a meaningful evaluation: one that describes the strengths, weaknesses, and potential exhibited by the student during this important assignment. This final evaluation is placed in the student's file and a copy is sent to the university placement office.

In most academic settings the university supervisor is responsible for assigning the final grade for the student teaching experience. Observation of the student's performance, assessment of written assignments, and the input and evaluation received by the master clinician form the basis for the grade assigned.

Clinical Hours

Supervisors are responsible for documenting the supervised clinical hours student clinicians accrue during the school practicum. A minimum number of contact hours with clients is required for state certification in the schools, American Speech-Language-Hearing Association Certification of Clinical Competence, and state licensure.

In some programs the master clinician maintains the record of practicum hours and signs these hours at the end of a successfully completed assignment. In other programs the university supervisor signs the hours that have been kept by the student clinician. An effective means of recording the hours is to devise one form that can be used for all clinical practica, both on and off campus. These forms should be in duplicate, and one set should be given to the student, and the other kept by the university. This insures the student accurate documentation when the time for verification of hours is needed. How grateful students are to have this information available! Stories abound from people seeking school certification, ASHA certification, or state licensing who find they are not able to verify their clinical hours because of lost personal copies, changes in university personnel, master clinicians who leave the field, and so forth.

Developing and Maintaining Public Relations

Good public relations promotes a mutual respect between school and university programs and establishes an effective communication system between the university supervisor and school personnel. It has been stated previously in this chapter that university supervisors have a responsibility to be a representative and liaison of the university program to the schools. Background in the schools gives supervisors an awareness of the importance of public relations in developing and maintaining effective communication between the university and school speech-language programs.

There are many benefits to be gained by the university when good public relations have been established, developed, and maintained:

1. School personnel are more inclined to provide the best possible experiences for a student clinician during the student teaching assignment. In all likelihood there will be a greater willingness on the part of school personnel to become involved in facilitating the experiential aspects of the student teaching program.

2. School personnel are likely to be more understanding of university procedures. When problems arise, they may extend additional cooperation to the university in helping to resolve them, such as the need for an extra master clinician and the need for special experiences.

3. School personnel probably will take a greater interest in working cooperatively with the university and will find a greater sense of satisfaction in maintaining a professional relationship.

4. Communication is enhanced; therefore, feedback to the university on the effectiveness of the student teaching program and the competence of student clinicians is facilitated.

5. A cooperative relationship encourages school personnel to share their program information and materials with the

university and, conversely, motivates university personnel to share innovations that are happening at the university level.

A supervisor contributes to public relations in many ways:

1. The supervisor knows and respects school protocol.
2. The supervisor knows etiquette appropriate for the schools and uses this knowledge judiciously.
3. The supervisor practices good manners, for example, when a supervisor schedules observations, it may be helpful to call in advance to alert the school staff to the planned visit. In addition, a brief visit with administrators, such as the principal, may gain support for the speech and language program. Expressions of appreciation to the appropriate personnel for services rendered does much to insure cooperative relationships with the schools.
4. The supervisor is quick to commend and slow to criticize school personnel, procedures, and activities.

CONCLUSION

Implementation of student teaching policies is a formidable and complex assignment. The combined efforts of the coordinator and supervisors are important if the university is to have a dynamic program, which commands the respect of student clinicians and school personnel.

The coordinator has many diverse responsibilities: organizing, disseminating information, contacting personnel, and acting as liaison between the university program and school districts. The supervisor also has many responsibilities that are inherent in the role of good supervision — observation, conferences, instruction, demonstration, and evaluation. Faculty chosen for this assignment should assume the role of supervisor-teacher, should observe student clinicians in the school setting, and should confer with them as they move through their school practicum.

When time and energy have been expended in developing an exemplary program, it is in the best interests of university faculty to maintain a cooperative relationship with the schools.

The efforts of the coordinator and supervisors can make student teaching one of the most meaningful and exciting experiences in the training program for all involved in the assignment. It brings to fulfillment the long period of preparation necessary for entry into the professional world. It is rewarding for faculty to guide their protégés through the final phase of their training program.

Chapter 10

PROSEMINAR

INTRODUCTION

Many training institutions provide student clinicians with a course pertaining to speech-language programs in the schools. Usually this is a requirement for students who plan to go into or who are presently in the student teaching program. In some institutions this course is taken prior to student teaching, while in other training programs, it is taken concurrently with the student teaching assignment. The purpose and content of the class will determine when students will enroll in such a course. Monnin and Peters discussed a course to be taken concurrently with student teaching, which "emphasizes implementation of specialized techniques, procedures for the public school setting, and the relations of language, speech and hearing services to the total educational program. Included within this structure are workshops conducted by selected master clinicians and guest speakers from the public schools on report writing, screening techniques, case selection and dismissal criteria, group dynamics, and other related topics" (1977, p. 102).

This chapter discusses a suggested course relevant to student teaching, Proseminar: Speech-Language-Hearing in the Schools. The course described delineates several areas that may be incorporated into a student teaching proseminar and is intended to serve as a guide for the instructor of such a course. The following description of a student teaching proseminar is not intended to be considered all-inclusive, nor will all the suggestions be applicable for every training program. It is expected that instructors of the proseminar will modify and adapt course content to meet the needs of their students and the standards established by their training programs.

A proseminar is defined as either an undergraduate seminar or graduate discussion group with fewer than twenty students. The format and activities of the course described are appropriate when students are enrolled concurrently in student teaching and small group interaction is desirable, beneficial, and constructive.

The basic purpose of the proseminar is to guide student clinicians through the student teaching experience; the emphasis is on the needs of student clinicians during this critical period in their training. The proseminar provides a structured contact with the training institution by bringing student clinicians to the campus on a weekly basis. In the student teaching assignment, student clinicians are separated from their peers and peer support. The proseminar provides regularly scheduled ongoing contact with university personnel and peers, which fulfills students' needs by being both supportive of their endeavors and informative of what is occurring in the field. The proseminar enables students sharing a common experience to come together to discuss their assignments and verbalize concerns as well as share information and pertinent suggestions. Group dynamics is an important feature of the proseminar. Through group interaction, various ways of managing the assignments are sought. Through awareness of group dynamics, student clinicians further their own abilities to work creatively with groups of pupils in the school assignment.

The proseminar provides opportunities for presenting topics of significant interest to student clinicians, such as federal and state laws affecting special education specifically in the area of speech-language pathology, admission and dismissal criteria of the case load, materials, therapy techniques, and interpersonal relations with school personnel. Student clinicians are encouraged to share materials they have used and found successful during their assignment. Journal articles and other publications pertaining to school speech-language programs may be discussed. Guest speakers may be invited to share information pertinent to working in the schools. Role playing may be used as a method for student clinicians to enact various roles they are called upon to fulfill.

The content of the proseminar is organized around the responsibilities of the speech-language pathologist in the school setting. As school program requirements change, so should the content of the proseminar. Input should be sought regarding educational trends from other university faculty members and school district personnel. When student teaching assignments encompass several school districts, student clinicians are exposed to a broad experiential base; therefore, the proseminar should be flexible enough to allow for discussion of intradistrict as well as interdistrict differences in programs, policies, and procedures.

It is recommended that faculty assigned to teach the proseminar be involved actively in the coordinating/supervising of student clinicians, thus providing current information and personal involvement necessary to make the proseminar a significant experience for the participants.

The composition of the class is limited to those students who are currently in student teaching. Scheduled as a weekly activity, students receive one or two units of university credit. Attendance is required, inasmuch as participation, not textbook knowledge, is the purpose of the proseminar. A midafternoon meeting time has proven expedient, freeing students to devote mornings and early afternoons to student teaching and evenings to other academic pursuits.

Grading practices will depend upon the university training program requirements: letter grade or credit/no credit. Using either method of grading, the instructor rates student performance on attendance, participation, completion of assigned activities, and overall competence displayed in the course.

The proseminar also provides practical preparation for professional employment in the schools. It is impossible to separate the immediate experiences of student clinicians from future professional performance, inasmuch as most of the requirements and information must, of necessity, be interrelated.

COURSE CONTENT

Architecturally, the proseminar is built on a four-pronged foundation: (1) lecture and discussion, (2) student activities, (3) student self-assessment, and (4) special events.

Lecture and Discussion

Federal and State Laws Affecting Education

Information on federal and state legislation should be discussed in the proseminar. Through lecture and outside readings, students will learn the significance of legislation and how it affects the speech-language pathologist in the school environment (Dublinske, 1978; Dublinske and Healy, 1978.) The specifics of legislation can be discussed in class, but competence in Individualized Education Programs, team conferences, and the assessment process can be achieved only through participation in those activities in the school setting.

Defining Educational Terminology

Each setting has terms that are appropriate for a special environment, and it is helpful if student clinicians learn these terms in conjunction with their assignments in the schools. Such terms as, PL 94-142, IEPs, DCH, RLS, SLD/A, TMR are meaningful for those working in particular educational settings. In the proseminar these terms can be discussed so student clinicians will be more knowledgeable about the school environment.

Ethical Practices

Ethical practices are defined as acts conforming to the standards of conduct of a given profession or group. One ethical practice that should be emphasized with student clinicians is confidentiality of information. Student clinicians should be aware of laws that protect pupils' privacy and be judicious about the information they share regarding pupils in the school case load. Although this may have been stressed in the on-campus clinic, it is important to remind student clinicians about their obligation to the pupils with whom they work.

The American Speech-Language-Hearing Association, state associations, and state licensure boards have established codes of ethics. Students must know their national and state codes, understand how they are protection for the consumer as well as the professional, and be prepared to adhere to them. Student clinicians should have copies of these codes before they move into work environments.

Interpersonal Relationships

Successful school speech-language pathologists attest to the necessity of establishing and maintaining effective public relations (PR). Laws can mandate, but unless the school speech-language pathologist strives to establish and maintain professional relationships and open lines of communication with others in the school environment, the speech-language program lacks a necessary component essential for success. Social amenities are important in professional relationships. Methods of achieving satisfactory interpersonal relationships with school personnel and the accompanying benefits can be explored with student clinicians in the proseminar setting.

Communication Aides

The use of supportive personnel is expanding, and student clinicians should know what the purpose of having communication aides is and how they function in the schools. Student clinicians need to understand how to work with communication aides and what the relationship is between professionals and paraprofessionals. Through lecture and readings, student clinicians will be better prepared to work with this group. Chapter 3 contains extensive information on students' relationships regarding the role and function of communication aides.

Videotapes

The adage "One picture is worth a thousand words" can be applied to videotapes used as demonstration in the proseminar. The instructor may wish to provide information on specific techniques used for therapy, ways to elicit responses from children, or means of stimulating group interaction. Showing videotapes of speech-language pathologists successfully using these procedures can have a greater effect and influence than lecture or reading assignments. The advantage of a taped session is that the instructor can emphasize specific points to be stressed. Viewers are exposed to the same stimuli, and there is consistency in what is seen each time the film is shown. In some cases the instructor may wish to show and discuss a particular tape when students begin the proseminar, and at a later date, after students have gained more practicum experience, they may be asked to critique the tape in order to demonstrate their growth in observation abilities.

Many training institutions have film libraries with well-stocked clinically oriented films. In some instances instructors may wish to develop a library of videotapes, emphasizing typical procedures used in the schools. A library of videotapes can be updated continuously as new information and techniques are introduced.

A recent development is *Telecourses,* which are available through the School Services Program of the American Speech-Language-Hearing Association (ASHA, 1977).

Selection of Materials

Now that students are providing services for more pupils with all types of speech and language disorders in an age range from preschool through high school, student clinicians need added sources for materials.

Students may need guidance in the selection and adaptation of materials to be used in the school setting. They should be advised on materials available from a variety of sources, such as commercial, programmed, second-hand articles, and computer games. Students need to know how to evaluate, modify, and use materials for specialized populations, such as the severe cerebral palsied and the developmentally disabled. There is a need to assess, adapt, and use materials appropriate for groups of children as well as for older pupils at the secondary levels. (Chapters 4 and 7 have suggestions for materials for older pupils.)

Capitalizing on Special Abilities

The proseminar can help student clinicians expand their therapeutic skills by encouraging them to utilize special abilities, such as singing, guitar playing, and creative dramatics. Student clinicians should be encouraged to draw upon their talents in order to realize their own potentials in creativity, as well as providing another therapeutic approach to foster communication skills in pupils seen in therapy.

Behavior Management

One major concern of student clinicians is management of group behavior. Most students have had some course background in group dynamics, but usually they have not had the practical experience of guiding pupils' behaviors in a group setting. The proseminar can help student clinicians learn how to work effectively with groups of children by helping them relate theoretical concepts acquired in previous course work to their current practicum experiences.

Students profit from discussions focusing on the advantage of group sessions, which may be more productive for some pupils than individual sessions. Frequently, student clinicians need guidance in using peer interaction to achieve the speech-language objectives established for each pupil. They need to become adept in group dynamics in order to learn how to avoid situations in which some pupils may receive too little attention and practice in group sessions. It is important for student clinicians to learn how to group pupils, when it is appropriate to do so, and when it is necessary to schedule individual therapy sessions. Age as a factor in this decision is discussed in Chapter 4.

Use of Equipment

In campus speech-language clinics, students have been introduced to the use of tape recorders, video equipment, Language Masters®, Phonic Mirrors®, and so forth as therapeutic aids. Student clinicians also should be cognizant of computer-age devices, such as electronic typewriters, language boards, voice machines, nonoral equipment for the severely handicapped, and other newly designed instruments. The availability, benefits, and uses of these aids can be discussed in the proseminar.

Problem Solving: Logistics

For the professional eager to perform competently, logistical breakdown is frustrating. Sometimes little things going wrong cause frustrations, which may result in student clinicians performing below their potential. Areas in which problems may occur are the following:

1. Getting the pupils to therapy and on time
2. Getting notations for one group written before the next group arrives
3. Having materials ready for the next group
4. Coping with last minute changes in school schedules
5. Getting information to classroom teachers and other school personnel

Although these areas are best handled in the practicum setting, the proseminar can give student clinicians alternatives and techniques to aid them in problem solving logistical breakdowns and maintaining a professional demeanor.

The preceding section of this chapter has addressed itself to several topics, which may be presented best through lecture and discussion. Some groups of students are eager to participate in open discussion, while other groups respond slowly to interacting among themselves and the instructor. In some cases students are reluctant to appear aggressive or are too unsure of themselves to take an active role in class discussion. Such students feel inadequate because of their perceived lack of experience and fail to recognize their potential as a contributing member in the proseminar. The discerning instructor will find methods to help them participate in group discussions.

A suggestion is to send a questionnaire to student clinicians and ask them to return it prior to the first class meeting. Students are asked to respond to questions, such as their experience working with children, talents they have developed, interests they wish to pursue, and goals they have for the future. Tabulate this information and hand out the results at the first class meeting. This approach reduces personal anxiety, as the class discussion focuses on a group profile rather than individuals. When the instructor recognizes and calls attention to students' experiences and talents, they find it more pleasant and rewarding than being called upon to report their own accomplishments.

The proseminar brings together for an extended period of time students who are undergoing a common experience, student teaching. Although they are having many basic similar experiences, there are differences unique to each assignment. The rationale for group discussion is its value as a learning experience in which students discuss and discover the value of different procedures, approaches, and experiences. Short answers to several topics and questions initiated by the instructor will generate discussion:

1. School district assigned
2. Number of master clinicians.
3. Assignment, i.e. elementary, intermediate, junior high, high school, special education site
4. Days assigned to student teaching.
5. Number of pupils in case load.
6. How much time spent observing *before* taking over case load.

7. How master clinician gives evaluation, i.e. oral/written.
8. When conferences with master clinician are scheduled, i.e. before school, after school, during lunch.
9. One word to describe the student teaching experience to date. To promote active involvement, have students use body movement to supplement their description. The purpose of this activity is to generate spontaneity of response.

Student Activities

Although lecture and discussion generate profitable learning experiences, the proseminar lends itself to other teaching modes. Some learning experiences are best achieved through direct student participation in assignments, such as observing, writing a philosophy, and compiling a materials bank. Through student activities the individual must assume responsibility for the practical application of theoretical knowledge.

Observations

Although student teaching introduces student clinicians to a work environment, it does not expose them to all the experiences available in the school setting. During the student teaching assignment, observations are a method for students to supplement their experiences and clinical skills by visiting other settings where speech-language pathologists are working with different populations, ages, and types of disorders. As students become more sophisticated clinicians, they also become more aware of the need for professional enrichment. Interacting with other speech-language pathologists, including those on special education sites and those with pupils from preschool through senior high school, provides valuable experiences by exposing student clinicians to the broad potentials of the school setting. Nationally, speech-language programs are most numerous at the elementary level (Schultz, 1972, p. 15); however, the schools offer many other programs with which students should be familiar. The proseminar provides a structured setting for assigning observations. In the proseminar, student clinicians derive added benefits from their observations by sharing, interacting, and discussing them with their peers. Suggested form may be found in the Appendix.

Reporting on District Procedures

Student clinicians may share information in the proseminar relative to screening procedures, data collecting practices, parent consent procedures, and admission and dismissal criteria used in their school districts. Interpretations of policies differ among school districts, and students may be surprised to discover the variations in procedures from one district to another.

Reading Assignments

In the proseminar, reading assignments are selected that relate specifically to the school setting: assessment techniques, therapy procedures, accountability, implementation of federal and state laws, use of paraprofessionals, role of the speech-language pathologist in educational settings, and so forth. The American Speech-Language-Hearing Association quarterly journal, *Language, Speech, and Hearing Services in Schools,* is a prime source of published articles directed toward the speech-language pathologist in the school setting.

Writing Skills

The implementation of federal laws requires speech-language pathologists to be efficient in writing Individualized Education Programs and long-range and measurable objectives for each pupil in the case load. The emphasis placed on writing lesson plans in the proseminar will depend on skills student clinicians have acquired previously. Student clinicians often need assistance in writing lesson plans for group therapy. They need instruction in planning group objectives, which incorporate the individual objectives for each pupil. They may also need guidance in implementing procedures that will aid in achieving both the individual and group objectives of the session. In helping students become more adept at writing lesson plans, the instructor may lecture, assign outside readings, conduct written exercises in class, or have students bring to class lesson plans they prepared or used in the schools. Any one or all of the foregoing procedures are enhanced when they are used for discussion by the class. The purpose of lesson plans is to clarify the objectives and therapeutic procedures for each pupil. Students should understand the purpose of lesson plans and place them in the proper perspective in order to attain the desired remediation results.

Every professional setting has established report writing standards. Students preparing for professional careers in the schools must develop and show general competence in writing ability as it pertains to school reports. The ability to express oneself clearly and unambiguously is becoming a lost art. The poor grammar skills and writing ability evidenced by today's youth is observed in every setting. It is ironical that as society requires a greater amount of paperwork, writing skills are declining. Practice in report writing can be incorporated into the various assignments in the proseminar. Competence and facility in writing should increase with practice. Students need to learn how to improve their writing ability, which is such a large part of their professional responsibility.

Presenting Case Studies

There are several situations in which students must be prepared to discuss pupils who evidence speech-language disorders, such as staffings with professionals from other disciplines to formulate appropriate recommendations and the admissions conference with parents and selected school personnel. Students will have had experience in discussing case studies in previous practicum assignments, but at this period in their training they should be capable of presenting in-depth case studies. Student clinicians may select one of the pupils in their case load and give a ten or fifteen minute presentation in the proseminar followed by class participation. When a particularly perplexing case is under discussion, group input can be beneficial in offering a wide range of suggestions or resolutions. Not only is this beneficial for the student who is presenting, but also it is informative for the others.

Sharing of Materials

An itinerant school speech-language pathologist often is required to move from one site to another in the course of a day. Materials should be compact, durable, and adaptable for different populations, age groups, and types of disorders. A suggestion for the instructor is to bring to class a small box filled with objects and demonstrate the variety of ways these materials can be used in therapy. A recommended group activity is to assign a project in which student clinicians present materials that are easily assembled, conveniently carried from one setting to another, and effectively used with different age levels. Through group discussion, ideas are generated for additional ways these materials can be used in therapy. Student clinicians enjoy selecting and sharing materials they have used successfully, and former students comment on the value of this segment of the proseminar.

An additional benefit of this project is that it provides an opportunity for student clinicians to speak before a group. Addressing oneself to peers is a difficult task; therefore, student clinicians should be expected to prepare a well-organized presentation using appropriate visual aids. A suggested evaluation form for this activity is included in the Appendix.

Organizing and Compiling an Information-Materials Bank

Most master clinicians generously offer materials that students may copy. Students collect handouts at workshops, conferences, and in-service meetings. The proseminar generates its own materials, and student clinicians collect catalogs and addresses of suppliers of therapy materials, along with information on books and articles that can be used in speech-language remediation. An activity that has proven highly successful is compiling and organizing a notebook and/or a jumbo letter file containing information and materials collected during the student teaching assignment. As a requirement of the proseminar, student clinicians are asked to categorize information that pertains to student teaching, e.g. schedules, information on pupils, lesson plans, comments from master clinicians and university supervisors, and self-evaluations of therapy sessions. Notes from the proseminar with information from guest lecturers and instructor are included. Student clinicians are asked to place in appropriate order materials that pertain to various types of speech-language disorders and various techniques that can be used for remediation. Some materials may be cross-referenced for use with several types of disorders. Therapy activities can be included in the file or mentioned in the notebook in a table of contents.

Requiring student clinicians to arrange this material in a systematic manner will be helpful, especially during their first year of professional employment when they have so many requirements on their time. This handy notebook or file will be a valued reference when planning implementation of therapy objectives.

Films

There are many excellent films that may be used as learning activities. These films, when shown in the proseminar, generate extensive discussion of their use and value in the therapeutic process. An example is the film *Tops* (Eames). It is especially appropriate for severe language handicapped pupils, as it has no narrative. It has been successfully used in the proseminar for writing lesson plans for a group of communicatively handicapped children. Discussions focus on the many different objectives that can be implemented through the use of this film, for example, articulation therapy, sequencing activities, categorizing, vocabulary building, and body movement. Through this presentation student clinicians can see how one film serves many speech-language purposes.

Student Self-Assessment

Ongoing self-assessment is essential if continued professional growth is to be realized. The time to train clinicians in self-evaluation is during the formative period when the student is in the educational program acquiring clinical skills. Self-assessment usually includes an evaluation of both professional skills and personal qualities.

Professional Skills

It is a highly valuable experience for student clinicians to assess formally their clinical strengths and weaknesses midway through their student teaching assignment and again at the conclusion of the assignment. Students should be aware of positive attributes they bring to student teaching as well as being able to identify changes that need to be made. A realistic self-assessment enables student clinicians to become more objective about their performance. When comparing midterm and final assessments, student clinicians will see the changes they have effected during this experience. The majority will feel a sense of personal achievement as they appraise their progress in student teaching. These assessments can also form the basis for conferences between the supervisor/instructor and the student clinicians. A suggested form is included in the Appendix.

Personal Qualities

To be able to look at oneself in an objective manner is a difficult assignment, even for the mature individual. The task of the training program is to help students evaluate the effectiveness or ineffectiveness of their personal qualities and behaviors for the profession they are about to enter. Qualities deemed necessary to be an effective and successful professional are discussed in Chapter 3. Areas of personal self-assessment include, but are not limited to, integrity, maturity, ability to accept instruction, adapt to changing situations, assume responsibility, and relate to pupils, peers, and adults. The proseminar can direct student clinicians' attention to personal qualities necessary for self-fulfillment in speech-language pathology as a helping profession.

A suggested way to promote interest, discussion, and worthwhile self-assessment in the proseminar is using The Keirsey Temperament Sorter, which is a similar but shorter form of the Myers-Briggs Types Indicator (Myers, 1962). The Keirsey Temperament Sorter is in the book, *Please Understand Me* (Keirsey & Bates, 1978), and provides a resource for self-assessment based on temperament styles developed by Jung (1923) in his description of function types.

Speech and Language Analysis

In addition to the preceding areas of self-assessment, a thorough speech and language analysis is important. Many master clinicians (Master Clinicians' Workshop, 1978) have requested that more attention be given to helping student clinicians analyze and monitor their speech, language, and vocal quality. Such factors as nasality, strident voice, articulation variations, pitch, vocal intensity, regional variations, vocabulary, and language structures have been suggested for inclusion in this assessment. Although regional variations may not cause concern in some areas, students should be able to modify regional patterns when appropriate. It is recommended that a speech and language analysis be a requirement of the proseminar. A suggested form may be found in the Appendix.

Statement of Philosophy: Speech-Language Services in the Schools

To define the role of the school speech-language pathologist, student clinicians need to understand the contribution of speech-language services within the context of the total educational program. How they define the role will determine to a great extent how they will function as professionals. There is no one philosophy that best defines their role; therefore, each speech-language pathologist will have a personal opinion of how the ideal program should function within a particular setting. Usually the school administrator or supervisor defines the district philosophy. It is helpful to student clinicians if they formalize a philosophy regarding their role as professionals. If they have a well-defined concept of their future role, they will be better able to seek employment in an environment that is compatible with their expectations.

Student clinicians have an opportunity during the proseminar to listen to and react to ideas presented by other members of the class. Examples follow that demonstrate the diversification of philosophies student clinicians have developed:

> Communicative abilities are important to one's academic success and psychological well-being. Our role is to aid children with speech-language disorders so that they may function better communicatively in the school environment and in the world at large.

> Providing speech-language services in the school is appropriate because it applies learning of speech-language behaviors in an environment rich in learning. What better place to provide communication experiences than in a setting focusing on learning?

> It is in the schools where a child's academic skills are learned. Success is dependent upon optimum speech-language skills. Speech-language remediation gives children experiences and opportunities to build for academic success.

> Since a major focus of childrens' lives occur in the public school, this is a unique and appropriate setting in which to undertake therapy. Children receive therapy in a natural and familiar environment that is usually supportive of their needs.

> I feel that the purpose of speech-language therapy is to help children achieve greater command of their environment so they can fulfill their needs through appropriate interaction with other people.

> My goal is to help children understand and communicate to their fullest potential so that they may in turn be better understood by the rest of the world.

> We, as speech-language pathologists, are God's helpers for those who cannot hear, cannot understand, cannot respond. We help create a communication process where it never existed or where it once flourished and was lost. We are at the beginning always, but never at the end. We are an important part of God's plan.

Formulating a statement of philosophy encourages students to think about their future role. In addition, personnel committees frequently ask interviewees for a philosophy regarding the place of speech-language services in education. The development of a philosophy prepares students to respond to this question during an employment interview.

Overview of Student Teaching Assignment

Before the assignment is concluded, it is advantageous for student clinicians to review their student teaching in its entirety. As the experience draws to a close, it is useful for them to step back from their immediate involvement in the assignment and review what activities they have participated in and accomplished in the school setting. Student clinicians often become so deeply involved in the day-to-day requirements they are unable to see the experience in its totality. By reviewing the interdependence of all the parts, student clinicians are forced to assess their experience from a holistic point of view. The advantage of writing an overview is that it forces students to evaluate the experiences they had and be aware of those activities in which they did not participate. Student clinicians may need to be reminded that it is impossible for them to participate fully in all the school activities in a limited period of time. A novice clinician can absorb only a finite amount of information during a given experience. Some of the experiences to which they have been exposed, but have not reached competence, are professional attributes to be developed in the future. A written overview of this important clinical practicum forces students to gain a realistic perspective of the assignment from its inception, the first day, to the last hurrah, its completion. An overview is a point of reference that may be used to measure other professional learning experiences.

This overview of the student teaching assignment, written by the student clinician, may be used by the university coordinator and supervisors to evaluate the effectiveness of the placement, on-site personnel, and experiences provided. It is a means of assuring the university that the student teaching requirements have been fulfilled.

In some training programs students submit a written evaluation of the master clinicians' effectiveness as cooperating training clinicians. Many institutions have a procedure for student evaluations of instructors. In these institutions an evaluation of master clinicians' performance would be consistent with university policy. However, master clinicians and student clinicians are not unanimous in supporting this evaluation procedure. Some master clinicians feel anxious and defensive about their role, and some student clinicians are concerned about the absence of anonymity, particularly if they will be working together as colleagues at a later date. The decision to use evaluations of master clinicians must, therefore, be made by the faculty of each training program.

Special Events

Another instructional mode that enriches the learning experiences offered in the course is special events. These may include guest lecturers, field trips, demonstrations of therapy techniques, in-service meetings, and so forth.

Guest Lecturers

Guest lecturers bring to the proseminar specialized information, particular interests, or individualized talent. Although the instructor selects and invites the guest lecturer, student clinicians may recommend particular individuals or request information on specialized topics.

Field Trips

Field trips allow student clinicians as a group to visit special settings for experiences not available on campus. This may include visiting settings with specialized facilities, visiting programs with specialized equipment and materials, or observing innovative therapy techniques. These experiences give students the opportunity to become directly involved with new materials, special equipment, and distinctive populations.

Workshops

Workshops provide special opportunities to bring student clinicians, master clinicians, and university faculty together to share a common experience. Topics for presentation are chosen that are of mutual interest to student clinicians and master clinicians.

Presenters may be current master clinicians, student clinicians, or other speech-language pathologists. Workshops also make it possible for those attending to meet the other student clinicians and master clinicians who are part of the student teaching program.

Workshops may be scheduled for a late afternoon or a Saturday morning when the participants can be together for an extended period of time. As a special event they may take the place of a regularly scheduled class meeting of the proseminar.

Workshops are the specific responsibility of the coordinator of student teaching (see Chap. 9); however, they usually are more responsive to the needs of the participants when the planning reflects the combined efforts of the coordinator, supervisors, and instructor of the proseminar.

District In-Service Meetings and State Conferences

Many large districts provide in-service meetings in which student clinicians may gain valuable information on techniques, procedures, and programs used within the district. Student clinicians should be encouraged to share information gained from these in-service meetings in the proseminar.

Student clinicians also should be encouraged to attend regional and state conferences. At these conferences they will be sharing a professional experience with a large number of speech-language pathologists from a variety of settings. As an added bonus, student clinicians learn about employment opportunities and job expectations as they mingle with the conference participants.

CONCLUSION

Students engaged in a common off-campus practicum experience, student teaching, come together to learn how to refine and expand the skills they are developing in the school setting. The proseminar enables students to meet with an instructor and with their peers to discuss among themselves their experiences in the schools. Faculty play an important role in student teaching by offering professional guidance and assistance. It is, however, important for students to discuss with each other their anxieties, joys, disappointments, and triumphs. The kinship of fellow students is a natural part of any academic endeavor; however, when students are physically separated from each other and the familiar academic environment, the need to share and compare takes on an added importance in their lives.

The proseminar provides unique opportunities for incorporating a variety of teaching modes, diversified activities, and student participation. It provides teaching opportunities for the instructor that are challenging and stimulating. Through discussion the instructor can help students learn the value of their opinions and appreciate their self-worth as they discover others listening to them and evaluating their comments, not as naive students, but as student clinicians about to bear the title Professional Speech-Language Pathologist.

Student activities enable the instructor to view and evaluate the total student—academician and clinician. During the major portion of the training program, university faculty see students performing either in academic courses or clinical practicum. The proseminar, by combining both academics and implementation activities, makes it possible for the instructor to observe how effectively the student incorporates and relates academic concepts to practical application for attaining therapeutic objectives.

The instructor is aware that most student clinicians are entering that point in their lives when peer relationships are changing from students-in-training to practicing professionals. When special events are scheduled, the instructor can observe the emerging maturity of student clinicians as they participate in activities and mingle with experienced professionals.

Probably the most rewarding experience for the instructor of the proseminar is observing the change in students throughout the time the class meets. During these months student clinicians move through the stages of dependency within the group to become independent professionals. For example, at the beginning of the course, students at *stage one* ask specific questions or make comments beginning with, "My master clinician says..." *Stage two* emerges when students say, "I would like to..." Students have entered *stage three* when they say, "I'm ready to..."

The instructor literally can watch *professionals* developing in a class once composed entirely of *students.* Midway through the course, subtle changes in physical behaviors can be observed. Student clinicians' behaviors are becoming more like professional clinicians. They walk, talk, and act the role they are portraying. They show confidence, joy, and security in what they are doing. They are moving confidently in the school environment and are emerging professionals in their own right. The greatest rewards an instructor can enjoy are to see growth in students, to guide them in assuming their professional responsibilities, and to prepare them for leadership roles in the profession. The proseminar is one course in which the individual entities of the training program merge to form the final gestalt.

APPENDIX
SUGGESTED FORMS

GUIDELINES FOR MASTER CLINICIANS

When practicing speech-language pathologists in the schools agree to assume the role of master clinicians, the question most frequently asked of the training institution is, "What do you want us to do?" In response to this question, I am suggesting guidelines that may aid you in implementing our mutual goals.

The student assigned to your supervision is a novice clinician who has had experience in the University Speech-Language Clinic performing therapeutic services primarily with clients on a one-to-one basis. There are many experiences that only the school environment can provide; therefore, student teaching is not giving a student more clinical experiences only but it is an integral part of the basic training necessary to convert a novice clinician into a competent clinician.

The following guidelines and suggestions are based on recommendations from master clinicians and former student clinicians. It is highly desirable for students to have experiences in several areas:

A. Identification and evaluation of children with possible speech, language, and hearing problems.
  1. Screening
    a. Experience with both group and individual screening
    b. Administering a variety of assessment procedures for children with problems in language, articulation, voice, fluency, and hearing impairments
  2. Selecting the case load; deciding which children—
    a. Will be enrolled in the speech-language program
    b. Do not qualify for speech-language therapy at this time
  3. Scheduling
    a. Criteria used for scheduling individual therapy
    b. Criteria used for grouping
    c. Factors determining number of children in a group
B. Conducting therapy for children with speech, language, and hearing problems

1. Establishing goals and objectives in accordance with federal and state legislation
2. Conducting therapy at various grade levels
3. Experience with various types of communication disorders: articulation, voice, language, dysfluencies, hearing impaired
4. Opportunity to evaluate children's achievement in therapy
    a. Evaluate results of each therapy session
    b. Evaluate periodically all children in therapy
5. Involvement in activities related to terminating therapy
    a. Criteria used for dismissing children
    b. Implementing carry-over by other persons, e.g. classroom teachers, parents
C. Conferring with families and other professionals regarding specific children, e.g. classroom teachers, school health personnel, school psychologist, guidance personnel, principal, vice-principals
D. Program administration
    1. Scheduling speech-language sessions with consideration for the total school program
    2. Preparing and maintaining records
    3. Compiling district and state reports
E. Relating to other school personnel and to the entire community in behalf of the speech, language, and hearing program; master clinicians should be alert to opportunities to demonstrate and discuss activities related to maintaining school and community relationships.

Student clinicians sometimes are unsure of the master clinician's philosophy. They need to know whether the master clinician expects them to follow a specific approach or whether they are to develop their own. Students recently have been exposed to various therapeutic methods, which may be different from those used by the master clinician, and student clinicians may need assurance that it is permissible for them to try a variety of approaches.

It has been found that student clinicians profit from close supervision and specific suggestions by master clinicians in these areas: planning appropriate goals and objectives, procedures to implement goals and objectives, therapy appropriate for attaining goals and objectives, selecting and using materials, group dynamics, and evaluating therapy sessions. Lesson plans are valuable because they require a student clinician to clarify goals and objectives and assess the means necessary to attain them.

If there is an indication of a weakness or an area of concern in the performance of a student clinician, do not hesitate to contact the university supervisor. Training a student to become a competent clinician is a coordinated effort involving many persons. Working out small difficulties early may alleviate larger problems from developing later.

Student clinicians start their student teaching with enthusiasm and anxiety. To allay the anxiety and encourage the enthusiasm requires understanding and professionalism from the master clinician.

Your student clinician, the university, and the profession are indebted to you for your invaluable aid in training future speech-language pathologists.

Coordinator, Student Teaching

GUIDELINES FOR STUDENT CLINICIANS

Student teaching is the culmination of many months, perhaps several years, of training and preparation. This part of your training is designed to develop your proficiency as a speech-language clinician in a working environment. Many persons are involved in providing you with this experience: university personnel, district supervisors, and master clinicians. These professionals are interested in helping you realize your potential as a competent speech-language clinician. It is hoped that student teaching will be an exciting and rewarding experience for you.

Student teaching is part of your total training; as such, it is expected this will be an opportunity for many learning experiences. You are not expected to be a polished speech-language clinician at this stage but, rather, a novice speech-language clinician who will gain proficiency as a result of this assignment.

Your primary responsibility at this time in your training is to your student teaching assignment. This is an exacting assignment, which will require a great deal of your time and energy. It is necessary for you to allow sufficient time in your academic and work schedules for the many demands that may be placed upon you, such as opportunities to attend in-service meetings, district staffings, and school conferences.

Following is information you will need to keep in mind as you proceed through student teaching.

1. Specific to the student teaching assignment:
   a. Beginning date _____
   b. Ending date _____
   c. School(s) assigned _____
   d. Master clinician(s) _____
   e. University supervisor _____
2. Grading procedures (e.g. pass/fail, credit/no credit, letter grade)
3. Some specific responsibilities to the student teaching assignment are as follows:

a. Adhering to the public school calendar and schedule
b. Lesson planning and record keeping
c. Conferring
   (1) Master clinician(s)
   (2) University supervisor
   (3) School personnel and parents
d. Establishing interpersonal relationships
e. Maintaining appropriate conduct, e.g. grooming, ethical practices, punctuality
f. Selecting, preparing, and utilizing materials
g. Demonstrating expressive and written competence
h. Demonstrating diagnostic and therapeutic competence
i. Self-assessing performance, i.e. growth, resourcefulness, strengths and weaknesses, dependability, maturity

You will feel some excitement and anxiety on the first day of your student teaching assignment. This is to be expected when you begin a new experience. Keep in mind your master clinician was a student clinician at one time and also experienced a first day in a new setting.

Coordinator, Student Teaching

OBSERVATION FORMAT

Student clinician's name_____
Session _____Date_____

1. Describe techniques or methods of therapy used.

2. Describe materials used.

3. What is the objective or purpose of each activity?

4. What is the relationship of the activity to the I.E.P.?

5. Describe significant behaviors noted (physical and verbal).

6. Make suggestions for follow-up lessons.

STUDENT CLINICIAN SELF-ASSESSMENT SUPPLEMENT

1. List your strengths and weaknesses as a student clinician.

   Strengths   *Weaknesses*

2. List ways you use your strengths to increase your competence as a student clinician.

3. List ways you will eliminate or minimize your weaknesses.

4. What do you consider a unique contribution you bring to your student teaching assignment?

5. Briefly describe ways you have changed or improved since your last self-assessment.

SPEECH TAPE CRITIQUE

Self-Analysis

Analyze your voice as though you were doing an in-depth diagnostic on a client. Evaluate each of the qualities listed below and cite evidence from the literature to support your conclusions.

Student _____ Date _____

Recording Environment _____

NASALITY	
ARTICULATION	
RATE	
VOCAL RANGE AND INFLECTION	
FLUENCY	
PITCH	

VOLUME	
INTERJECTION	
DIALECT/ ACCENT	
QUALITY	

Comments _____

_____

_____

_____

_____

References _____

_____

_____

_____

_____

Student

ORAL PRESENTATION

Rating   *Areas to be Evaluated*

_____ Organization of presentation

_____ Knowledge of the topic

_____ Ability to give adequate background information and then develop the topic to a level that is appropriate for a proseminar

_____ Ability to select and present the most salient parts of the project

_____ Ability to evaluate material presented and draw relevant conclusions

_____ Ability to present material in a clear, concise, understandable way

_____ Manner of presentation, i.e. reliance on notes, eye contact, poise

_____ Ability to respond to questions

_____ Depth of research of the topic

_____ Bibliography: academic level and appropriateness of references

_____ Overall presentation

Comments:

COMMUNITY COLLEGE
SPEECH–LANGUAGE INTAKE FORM

Name _____

Address _____
                Street   City   Zip

Telephone _____ Social Security No. _____

Date of birth _____ Place of birth _____

Native language _____

Academic major or vocational goal _____
_____

Speech-language problem _____
_____
_____
_____

   * * * To be filled in by Speech-Language Pathologist * * *

Speech-language diagnosis _____
_____
_____

Recommendations _____
_____
_____

COMMUNITY COLLEGE SPEECH–LANGUAGE CLINIC REFERRAL RESPONSE FORM

To: Date:

From: Speech-Language Pathologist

_____ (Student's name) _____ has come for a speech-language interview.

_____ S/He will be scheduled for a diagnostic evaluation.

_____ S/He has been scheduled for a diagnostic evaluation.

_____ S/He has chosen to defer speech-language therapy at this time.

_____ Speech-language therapy was not recommended.

Comments:

REFERENCES

1. Anderson, J.: Supervision of school speech, hearing, and language programs — an emerging role. *ASHA, 16:*7–10, 1974.
2. ASHA, Committee on Speech and Hearing Services in the Schools: Recommendations for housing of speech services in the schools. *ASHA, 11:*181–182, 1969.
3. ASHA, Committee on Supportive Personnel: Guidelines for the employment and utilization of supportive personnel in audiology and speech-language pathology. *ASHA, 23:*165–169, 1981.
4. ASHA, Committee on Supportive Personnel: Guidelines on the role, training, and supervision of the communication aide. *Speech Hearing Serv Schools, 2:*48–53, 1970.
5. *ASHA,* The School Services Program, Telecourses. *Lang Speech Hearing Serv Schools, 8:*69–71, 1977.
6. Backus, O.: Group structure in speech therapy. In Travis, L. (Ed.): *Handbook of Speech Pathology,* 1st ed. New York, Appleton-Century-Crofts, 1957, pp. 1025–1064.
7. Bailey, R.: Why I quit. *New York Times, 33,* July 30, 1975.
8. Black, M.: *Speech Correction in High Schools.* State of Illinois, Office of the Superintendent of Public Instruction, 1960.
9. Breakey, L., Kesterson, S., Price, B., and Rasmussen, L.: Community colleges and the speech pathologist. California Speech and Hearing Association ad hoc committee report presented at California Speech and Hearing Association Annual Convention, March 27, 1977, San Francisco, California.
10. Breakey, L., Price, B., Rasmussen, L., and Zeller, E.: A model comprehensive plan for speech pathology programs in the community colleges. Consortium Report, 1978. (Photocopy.)
11. Caracciola, G., Morrison, E., and Rigrodsky, S.: Supervisory relationships and the growth in clinical effectiveness and professional self-esteem of undergraduate student clinicians during a school based practicum. *Lang Speech Hearing Serv Schools, 11:* 118–126, 1980.
12. Cartwright, D., and Zander, A.: *Group Dynamics: Research and Theory.* New York, Harper & Row, 1960.
13. Chapey, R., Burke, J., Schiavetti, N., Denson, T., and Lubinski, R.: Survey of language, speech and hearing services at community colleges. *ASHA, 19:*470–472, 1977.
14. Community Colleges Chancellor's Office: *Handbook: Guidelines for Community College Speech-Language-Hearing Programs.* Mr. Robert Howard, Special Services Unit, Community Colleges Chancellor's Office, Sacramento, California, in press.

217

15. *Conference on Standards for Supervised Experience for Speech and Hearing Specialists in Public Schools.* Orange County Department of Education, Santa Ana, California, 1969.
16. Culatta, R., and Helmick, J.: Clinical supervision: the state of the art, Part I. *ASHA, 22:*985–993, 1980.
17. Dublinske, S.: Special reports: PL 94–142: developing the Individualized Education Program (IEP). *ASHA, 20:*380–397, 1978.
18. Dublinske, S., and Healey, W.: PL 94–142: Questions and answers for the speech-language pathologist and audiologist. *ASHA, 20:*188–205, 1978.
19. Eames, C.: *Tops.* Produced by the University of Southern California, Los Angeles, California, 7 minutes, color film.
20. Gage, M.: Personnel, Division of Special Education, Los Angeles City Unified School District, Los Angeles, California. Personal communication.
21. Gottlieb, B.: Incidence of speech and language problems at Cerritos College. Unpublished, 1967.
22. Halfond, M.: Clinical supervision—stepchild in training. *ASHA, 6:*441–444, 1964.
23. Hayes, T.: Case selection in secondary schools. *The Voice,* 22 – 23, Feb. 1969.
24. Jung, C.: *Psychological Types.* New York, Harcourt Brace, 1923.
25. Keirsey, D., and Bates, M.: *Please Understand Me: An Essay on Temperament Styles.* Del Mar, California, Prometheus Nemesis Books, 1978.
26. Lewin, K.: *Field Theory in Social Science.* New York, Harper, 1951.
27. Leonard, M.: Introducing student teachers to group therapy. Oral presentation at Master Clinician/Student Teacher Workshop, Professionally Speaking, Feb. 1976, Los Angeles, California.
28. Leonard, M.: Seminar on speech therapy on the secondary level. Lecture presented at California State University, Los Angeles, May 1975.
29. Maltz, M.: *Psycho-Cybernetics.* New York, Simon & Schuster, 1960.
30. Marge, M.: The gift of speech. *American Education,* U.S. Department of Health, Education and Welfare, Office of Education, Nov. 1965.
31. Master Clinicians Workshop. Sponsored by California State University, Los Angeles, Feb. 1978.
32. Miami, Florida: *Miami-Dade Community College, 1979-1981 Catalog,* vol. 19, no. 1, 1979.
33. Monnin, L., and Peters, K.: Problem solving supervised experience in the schools. *Lang Speech Hearing Serv Schools, 8:*9–106, 1977.
34. Murphy, A.: Stuttering therapy and the personal psychology and philosophy of the clinician. Paper presented at the American Speech and Hearing Association Annual Convention, Las Vegas, Nevada, Nov. 5–8, 1974.
35. Myers, I.: *The Myers-Briggs Type Indicator.* Princeton, Educational Testing Service, 1962.
36. Neidecker, E.: *School Programs in Speech-Language: Organization and Management.* Englewood Cliffs, Prentice-Hall, 1980.
37. Offer, D.: *The Psychological World of the Teenager.* New York, Basic Books, 1969.

38. Oratio, A.: *Supervision in Speech Pathology: A Handbook for Supervisors and Clinicians.* Baltimore, University Park Press, 1977.
39. O'Toole, T.: Supervision of the clinical trainee. *Lang Speech Hearing Serv Schools,* 4:132–139, 1973.
40. O'Toole, T., and Zaslow, E.: Public school speech and hearing programs: things are changing. *ASHA,* 11:499–501, 1969.
41. Palmer, M.: Speech disorders of childhood. *Feelings,* Ross Laboratories, Columbus, Ohio, vol. E #3, March 1964.
42. Pasadena, California, Pasadena Area Community College District. *Bulletin of Pasadena City College: A Public Two Year Community College District,* April 1980.
43. Peters, K.: Survey of speech-language-hearing programs in Florida community colleges. Unpublished, 1980.
44. Polite, J.: In-service isn't really education. *Today's Education,* 69:35GS, Nov.–Dec. 1980.
45. Ratkevich, T.: Seminar on speech therapy at the secondary level. Lecture presented at California State University, Los Angeles, March 1975.
46. Scalero, A.: The use of supportive personnel in a public school speech and language program. *Lang Speech Hearing Serv Schools,* 7:150–158, 1976.
47. Schubert, G.: *Introduction to Clinical Supervision in Speech Pathology.* St. Louis, Warren H. Green, Inc., 1978.
48. Schultz, M.: *An Analysis of Clinical Behavior in Speech and Hearing.* Englewood Cliffs, Prentice-Hall, 1972.
49. Smith, G., Wagner, C., and Lopez, T.: The prevalence of speech disorders in a community college student population. Unpublished, 1976.
50. Vairo, P., and Perel, W.: Preparation of the cooperating teacher. *The Clearing House: A Journal for Modern Junior and Senior High Schools.* 48:131–134, 1973.
51. Van Hattum, R.: *Clinical Speech in the Schools.* Springfield, Thomas, 1969.
52. Van Riper, C.: Supervision of clinical practice. *ASHA,* 7:75–77, 1965.
53. Willbrand, M., and Tibbits, D.: Compensation for supervisors of clinical practicum in public school settings. *Lang Speech Hearing Serv Schools,* 7:128–131, 1976.

INDEX